Early Relational Trauma and the Development of the Self

Through the attentive examination of a single case study, this book weaves together the lived experiences of a clinician in training with those of their teenage patient, as they collectively navigate and overcome the profound effects of early relational trauma on the development of the self.

By the care taken in their analysis, the book's authors deepen readers' understanding of attachment disorders and their clinical presentation whilst allowing for a uniquely human view of the interactions between patient and clinician. Elegantly combining poetic prose with a clinical account, this book invites readers to travel with the clinician, to think and feel in tandem with his subjective experiences, and to explore psychoanalytic and systems theory as a means to understand clinical relationships that are seldom written about with such vulnerability. It is a story of determination and growth both moving and enlightening.

By giving form to the resilience of both patient and clinician, their mutual strength through "tears of change", this book expounds the behavioral consequences and treatment of psychopathologies associated with early relational trauma. In this way, the book will prove essential for all psychoanalysts and psychotherapists working with traumatized children and adolescents.

Tomás Casado-Frankel (Author) is faculty and supervisor in the Child & Adolescent Psychotherapy Training Program at the William Alanson White Institute. He is a graduate of that program and its psychoanalytic program. He coauthored *Psychological Aspects of Deportation and Child Custody*, a chapter in Appleseed's online manual, *Protecting Assets and Child Custody in the Face of Deportation.* He is also a graduate of the Couple & Family Therapy program at the Universidad Pontificia Comillas, in Madrid, Spain, and holds a postgraduate diploma in Conflict & Dispute Resolution Studies from Trinity College Dublin, in Ireland. He is in private practice in New York City.

María Eugenia Herrero MD and PhD (Author) holds specialties in Psychiatry (Madrid), Forensic Psychiatry (Madrid), and Family Psychotherapy (Tavistock Clinic/San Pablo CEU, London & Madrid). She founded "Project Sirio" in 1998, and was the director of its two therapeutic communities for twenty-two years. Project Sirio is a pioneering therapeutic community for children and adolescents with severe mental health problems, who are under the legal custody of the Government of Madrid. It is a team of 40 professionals, including psychiatrists, psychologists, social workers, teachers, and art therapists. The Project treats children and adolescents, most of whom have histories of severe neglect and/or abuse, and who have attachment difficulties and disorders, and exhibit or are at serious risk of developing borderline traits, or full-fledged BPD. Dr. Herrero is former Honorary Professor of the Department of Psychiatry of the Autónoma University of Madrid, and a Member of the Task Force on Child Maltreatment and New Models of Child and Youth Mental Health Treatment of the Council of Health of the Madrid Government. She has given Conferences, Seminars, and Workshops in a number of Spanish Hospitals and Schools of Medicine and Psychology on topics related to Attachment Disorders. In addition to being the clinical supervisor of the psychotherapists who work with children and their families in Project "Sirio", Dr Herrero has recently developed two further initiatives: One directed to support and accompany young mothers with BPD and related psychopathologies, who suffered severe neglect or abuse as children (a Mother-Child Dyadic Group); the other to help post-adolescents with BPD subsequent to their underlying attachment disorders, to build better ways to integrate in work and social life. Dr. Herrero is deeply committed to breaking the stigma of mental illness.

Pascal Sauvayre (Editor) is faculty, training, and supervising analyst at the William Alanson White Institute, he writes and studies at the interdisciplinary boundaries of psychoanalysis, recent projects include the co-editorship of *The Unconscious: Contemporary Refractions in Psychoanalysis* (Routledge, 2020), and current projects include the translation of Jean Laplanche's *The Tub: The Transcendence of the Transference* at The Unconscious in Translation, and co-editorship of *Breaking Boundaries: Culture, Gender, and Race in the Making of Interpersonal Psychoanalysis* (Routledge, forthcoming), and he has a private practice in New York City.

Early Relational Trauma and the Development of the Self

A model of therapeutic accompaniment

Tomás Casado-Frankel and
María Eugenia Herrero

Edited by Pascal Sauvayre

Translated from Spanish by
Tomás Casado-Frankel

Routledge
Taylor & Francis Group

LONDON AND NEW YORK

Cover image: Daniel Sánchez de Miguel

First published 2022
by Routledge
4 Park Square, Milton Park, Abingdon, Oxon OX14 4RN

and by Routledge
605 Third Avenue, New York, NY 10158

Routledge is an imprint of the Taylor & Francis Group, an informa business

© 2022 Tomás Casado-Frankel and María Eugenia Herrero

British Library Cataloguing-in-Publication Data
A catalogue record for this book is available from the British Library

Library of Congress Cataloguing-in-Publication Data
A catalog record has been requested for this book

ISBN: 978-1-032-19912-2 (hbk)
ISBN: 978-1-032-19932-0 (pbk)
ISBN: 978-1-003-26149-0 (ebk)

DOI: 10.4324/9781003261490

Typeset in Times New Roman
by MPS Limited, Dehradun

First and foremost, for the children.

And for all those who would like

to learn how to accompany them.

Contents

Yao Lu

A long time ago now, on a sunny autumn day, from a distant country, Yao Lu cut through the skies aboard a gigantic airplane, and made her way to Spain. She was only eight or nine.

In the complex and diverse society of Spain of the time, Yao Lu landed in a single-parent family: with a mother and no father. With three grown daughters of her own, Amalia, her adoptive mother, dared to take another child under her wing after overcoming diverse financial, and health-related problems, and after having successfully put her elder daughters «on the right track» as she put it. She was a prototypically conventional functionary but with a trendy touch as expressed in her use of new technologies and the way she proudly drove her classic (not old) car, which took her around everywhere. She strove to impose order and discipline in her home and family, as she monitored the development of each of her daughters under the scrutiny of her silvery blue eyes, obsessively repeating her wish that they study, so that they could eventually make a living of their own.

And yet Yao Lu, slender and supple as a reed, even taller than her rather large mother, stood in stark contrast to her. With her deep and penetrating gaze, she seemed to escape her mother's grasp. They both loved one another, and made an effort to understand each other, but were only partially successful. They were not in sync.

Yao Lu remembered very little about her biological mother. Of her biological father, she remembered more: the pail of dirty water where he had repeatedly tried to drown her, the strokes of the green bamboo canes on her frail little-girl legs, and the still sharp scars on her ankles, left by the ropes he used to bind her, when he would hang her upside down. Then came the long years in orphanage, hard years also, but happier. Then Amalia arrived in her life.

After living in Spain with her single-parent family for many years, Yao Lu was placed in the unconventional family of Sirio, the Therapeutic Community, which took her in to treat her psychological problems. It was there, always with the aim of healing, that the work on reattachment and accompaniment took place. She lived in the Community with eight other adolescents. As was the case with each of her peers, she was assigned a professional educator. Javier was a part of a whole team, working with her in her daily life, through her lived experiences, her life difficulties and her very troubled and complex relationships.

Yao Lu arrived from a rural corner in China, and this is a fragment of the life story of the *girl who made her way from afar* to our globalized society of today. This book is but a small piece—much like the piece of a jigsaw puzzle—of the complex multidimensional treatment carried out by a large multidisciplinary team, devoted to child and adolescent mental health. Written in the first person, this is the narrative of the young therapeutic companion who stood beside Yao Lu during an eventful period of her life.

Yao Lu was an adolescent, an adopted daughter in a single-parent family; she initially arrived in Spain at the age of 8 or 9, following an international adoption process. She rapidly learned to speak Spanish— what a new universe emerging in her mind!—and she settled into school. She had a friendly smile, yet relationships with other children were always difficult and complex for her. And she soon began to experience—re-experience, as we discovered—abuse in our Western world.

Old wounds and unhealed injuries, unknown to her caretakers at that time, began to surface. She came to the attention of many health care professionals, received different psychological and medical treatments and therapies, but the family felt overwhelmed and confused by so many and so frequent problems... For months and years, and despite various highly qualified recommendations, stays at boarding schools, therapies, classes, and all sorts of treatments, her progress remained uneven and difficult at best.

One day, late in her teens, she landed at the doorstep of our Therapeutic Community with her large dark eyes and her gentle smile. From then on, she shared her life with us, her successes, but mostly her difficulties with family, school, and interpersonal relationships. This included ten months of a pregnancy she decided to carry through and the resulting postpartum period, during which she had to be referred to a specialized facility for young mothers. Later she returned to us, to our Therapeutic Community, until her final departure, close to her coming of age. Her life has gone on and the years have gone by.

Problems such as hers are all too common in our society, and feasible solutions to the complex difficulties of our children and adolescents are urgently needed. Time, ever so fleeting for all of us, goes by even more frenetically for them. And so this story needs to be told.

Who are "we"?

For Yao Lu we were her new surrogate family, when her own felt unable to care for her and to address her many needs. This is what we try to be for each and every one of the children we look after.

We are a multidisciplinary team, specializing in psychiatric treatment and therapeutic work with children and adolescents who exhibit serious mental health problems. They live with us for mid to long-term stays, where they are also under some measure of protection, due to situations involving various risk factors, including family violence, abuse, and neglect.

We are a large team, of close to 40 people organized into two small *therapeutic communities*—we call them *Homes*. In the US, the closest kind of facility is referred to as a long-term adolescent residential facility. Nine children and adolescents, both male and female, coexist and live together in each. These Homes provide individualized, specific, and global psychiatric treatment in all areas of the life and development of the child or adolescent: psychological, relational, educational, familial, social, academic, recreational and, when the time comes, vocational. Always attentive and open, we accompany them in their lives and needs, in their achievements and difficulties, never closing, 365 days a year. At the time, both in Madrid and in Spain, we were pioneers in this type of care and treatment of serious childhood and adolescent mental health disorders, especially *attachment disorders.*

A large team of experienced, eager, and active men and women—
psychologists, teachers, nurses, occupational therapists, sociologists,
etc.—led by a woman (in our case) psychiatrist-psychotherapist, live
with, accompany, and educate the children. The goal is to help these
children develop in our Community as in a large atypical family,
where they may find and experience the bonds and reparative and
reconstructive attachments with figures that many of them never had
and could never experience in their early lives. Through such
relationship they may reconstruct, or have a second chance to build,
the pillars of their personality and wounded psyche. That is the daily
bread of our work. Children who during the early stages of life have
lacked that affectional bond with a mother figure—a primary figure
and *secure base* for the pillars of a healthy personality with good
enough mental health—can reconstruct it and be able to experience it
with us. This work is what we call *re-attachment*.

As might be easily imagined, ours is thus a deep and detailed work,
a slow one, frequently arduous, that advances and falters, that inches
forward, getting our children to develop one step at a time, at their
own rhythm and pace. They are given the opportunity to develop
positive experiences in their mind-heart-body with a narrative that
may allow them to live and understand the world with a trusting eye,
or at least a less distrusting one.

Our children have what we could easily refer to as the *illness of
mistrust*. They are suspicious, disbelief etched in their eyes, fearing to
venture closer, always anticipating harm from the other, or mockery, if
not negligence, abuse, or maltreatment. That is what they have had to
live through during their first few years, with far too little of a nurturing
environment, and caretakers available to provide the compensatory
stability of trust and unquestioned security, necessary features for a
minimal state of harmony to be able to grow and construct themselves.
They have never been free from having to be constantly alert and tense,
on the lookout so as to ward off impending danger. Without the
experience of a parent's relaxed cradling arms, carrying them safely
with tenderness and care, caressing them with soft and gentle words
murmured into their ears, they have had to fend for themselves.
Instead, they have had to permanently be on the lookout for new and
lurking dangers visited on them arbitrarily, by the very parental figures
or caretakers they depend on, "care"takers who are negligent of the

child's basic needs, or seriously abusive or maltreating. All of the child's attention and focus has been devoted to not being attacked or assaulted, on sheer survival.

As a result, the habitual attitude of these kids is to be on the defensive, mistrustful, often attacking before being attacked themselves. *Serious difficulty in social relatedness, in interpersonal relations*, is therefore their biggest problem. This difficulty seeps into every other sphere of their lives. These are children without friends, with limited capacity for empathy. They approach relationships with little awareness and ability to negotiate boundaries, and they must face massive rejections. They lack friendships that could help them enhance their own identity (Kernberg et al. 2000). But many learn to want them, to seek them and to learn how to experience them.

Our ultimate goal is to allow them to achieve adequate social inclusion, to gain as much freedom and personal autonomy as possible, so that they can grow and develop *creative relationships* in the areas of love, friendship, work, and social life (Normandin et al., 2014). This can only take place when there is trust in the relationship, a basic trust, a foundational feeling of being accepted for simply being who they are, not for acting or pretending to be someone they are not. And this is difficult, very difficult.

Our task with the children and adolescents—like that of the "good enough" mother/father (Winnicott, 1971), who accompanies and tenderly educates the child with care—is like the artisan with his/her apprentice, experimenting with and transmitting values and behaviors by modeling. We provide the children an experience of what it is like to be sought after, accompanied, heard, valued. It is about the construction of healthy boundaries, so the child need not feel overwhelmed, and may feel *safe enough*. What we provide is much like what a mother does when she cares for and accompanies, but also respects, the child, who can then begin to experiment, explore, and make healthy and positive choices. The child can then learn from his/her own strengths and mishaps, while he or she feels the progressive increase in freedom, having broken the shackles of mistrust and failure that were a hindrance before. Our job with these children, therefore, is done in a place of uncertainty, in the difficult balance of choosing between safety and freedom, according to how far each child is on his/her own developmental trajectory, depending on their age and their personal circumstances in life.

This story is but one example of the kind of specific and tailored work we do, the story of Yao Lu, one of our female teenagers, and Javier, one of the educators on our team, the therapeutic companion who worked with her for over two and a half years, three times a week. He will be our narrator. For the project director it involved two and a half years of careful supervision, close communication, daily dialogue—over email, phone or face-to-face—provided at all hours of the day and night, through which Javier gradually constructed that reparative bond with Yao Lu, who, for diagnostic purposes, can be said to suffer from a severe and distorting *attachment disorder*, which crystallizes into borderline pathology with psychotic features.

The supervisory work per se is not addressed in our book. We have preferred to allow it to filter through the explanations and descriptions of the experiences woven together by Javier, that at least partially and progressively reveal the foundations of the theory that supports the daily ethos behind the work taking place in our therapeutic community. We are presenting just a part of the overall treatment that took place here: the accompaniment and reparative reattachment, which required creativity, hopefulness, a belief in Yao Lu's capabilities, and significant efforts from all of us.

After many meetings and diverse reviews and re-readings, we have decided that the tender and delicate tone of our story should be kept, though moderately mitigated, even though it could draw criticism and be deemed overly sentimental by the clinically objective reader. This is because, in addition to the clinical literature and scientific foundations that support our work, *the narrative envelope,* as referred to by Daniel Stern, permeates the daily reality of the work, with the use of loving voices and delicate words, as a mother might use with her baby. Yao Lu lacked that primary mother figure in her life and we had to make use of this second chance for her to experience it, to rebuild herself, and heal her deep psychic injuries. We had to work with enough empathy and consideration to create that necessary tenderness to fight against the dominance of a radical mistrust and the paranoid states of a girl that experienced and survived situations of severe psychic trauma. She was an adolescent who as a little girl had repeatedly experienced the «confusion of tongues between the adults and the child», where the boundaries between tenderness and passion disappear (Ferenczi, 1949), a confusion created by adult men in her case.

What might the goal of our story be then? What are the ideas we would like to convey throughout these pages? The following list identifies key aspects of what is a delicate tapestry of human relationships and their evolution:

1   *Early affective attachment* of the human infant with the mother (or surrogate caregiving figure), which takes place during the first stages of life, if it occurs under good enough conditions, *is a pillar and foundation for the mental health of the developing person.*

2   This *mental health encompasses many fundamental aspects of the human subject: the capacity for interpersonal relations, the intellectual and cognitive capacity to understand and decipher the world, the ability to adapt to environmental stressors with adequate social behavior as a manifestation of that health, and the balanced development of moral conscience itself.* Mental health, therefore, cannot solely be defined as the absence of psychic illness.

3   The healing of this absence/lack of this early affective bond, which has a variety of causes including negligence, parental mental illness, maltreatment, abuse, social difficulties or challenges in work-life balance, and scarce maternal presence or availability in the complex society of today, and its severe relational, cognitive, emotional, and behavioral sequelae,—is an arduous, costly, prolonged, and difficult, but not impossible, task. We call this healing *re-attachment.*

4   Many of the children adopted from distant lands, in addition to growing numbers in our society who present similar difficulties, are burdened by this harmful deficit that they carry in their tiny backpacks. It is in their baggage, yet rarely in their files or reports, when they arrive in Spain.

5   The parents and families who sought them, who await them, who wish for them and eagerly open their arms to them, should be supported and guided, as well as adequately selected and informed, in order to be able to take the complex and prolonged journey with their children to fruition. All parents need support, but these adoptive families may very likely need it more.

6   We would like to use this book to introduce you to part of our work on attachment and reattachment. This is the work we do in our Therapeutic Community; where a multi-professional team treats diverse children and adolescents who suffer from serious mental health problems, generally related to attachment. We also work with their families, when they exist, and in coordination with very diverse institutions related to childhood, and in the polyhedral, fast-paced, complex, and concrete, shifting social community of Madrid, we even hit the streets, as was the case with Yao Lu.

7   We would like our story to capture our experiences and make them useful for the many educators and parents who need and demand it from us, and urgently so. But we must take one step at a time, as we do in our daily work. We would therefore rather *like this to be a first step.* As an extension of our teamwork, we view the book as the beginning of a road towards the transmission and discovery of profound and important lessons in relation to early childhood. We are now ready to listen to and experience the telling of this tale. To live and listen to Yao Lu's life and that of her educator Javier, who accompanies her and who will provide the conceptual clarification of the underpinnings of the complex dynamics that structured her life day to day, a life which may have otherwise seemed simple.

This book is at once both simple and complex.

Apparently simple, because it narrates and relates snippets and moments in the life of our adolescent-girl—as Javier, her *therapeutic educator* calls her—over a period of more than two and a half years, and because it is he, the one chosen to carry out this job by our diligent multidisciplinary team, who speaks of the events.

Complex, not only because life is always complex, but also because Yao Lu's life, *our girl on the road from afar,* arrived from the East to her new family with her tiny backpack full to the brim with hidden and secret sufferings and enormous psychic injuries that could have even worsened here.

Complex, because during the three long years that are here described, Yao Lu progressed from an adolescent-girl to a mother, to an adolescent-woman who moved through times of dark despair, when death was near, sought out, wished for, even announced at times, to times where little glimmers of hope began to make their way into the darkness and provide a new horizon.

Complex too, because what this story speaks of is the construction of a reparative bond—perhaps a saving one—between a rejected, despised, maltreated, and utterly self-denigrating and belittled girl-mother, and a young male educator in training, full of hope, who with great ability and determination did what he could to rescue her as he himself developed professionally. He managed to understand and intuit the essence of the work that takes place in our Therapeutic Community of Project Sirio, which can be summarized thus: for Yao Lu to be able to heal, love, and believe in herself, it was first necessary that she could trust and establish a trustworthy relationship. And they had to create it *from scratch*.

In the long and arduous road of accompanying someone—almost three years seems like such a long time—this educator, under close and sustained supervision from his psychiatrist director, took strides in his own process of becoming self-aware, in his capacities and limitations, allowing himself to trust and grow with her, reconstructing and building her self-worth, while he studiously worked through each issue and obstacle that arose along the way, and which would shape his professional career.

We have tried to avoid overly detailed or predetermined explanations of the prior life of our girl—slightly fictionalized with names, dates, and locations modified to preserve her privacy—which might perhaps lead to prejudices and hasty conclusions on the part of the reader. Instead we invite you to listen carefully and attentively.

This book is therefore both dense and profound, technical, and colloquial, on the border of everyone's experience, in no-man's-land, and yet connected to all of us. It is precisely the field we work in. This is a story to learn a great deal from and to read slowly, a story which may be moving and touch you deeply.

Chapter 1

Introduction

1.1 Attachment disorder

During the 1980s and even in the 1990s, this serious childhood psychopathology was rarely, if ever, diagnosed in Spain. Pervasive inattention and the lack of resources and specialized services for the treatment of child and adolescent disorders was the norm, compared to the high quality of the rest of the medical specialties and pediatric services in Spain's medical field.

1.1.1 Naïve ideas of happy childhoods

The naïve and archaic belief about the early years, *all children are good and happy*, has been widespread in our community and society; and mental health problems, of whatever kind, were really considered to exist only in the adult population. If thought of at all, the general public believed that child and adolescent mental health consisted in treating children presenting with cognitive problems or intellectual disabilities. It was Nuevo Futuro, a non-profit organization, established in the legendary year of 1968, that fought to «break away the infantile chains»—much like Pinel in the adult French Salpêtrière, of the XVIII century—of the large hospices and orphanages, and that influenced the government and policymakers to change the obsolete Adoption Law, in order to allow for placing children in small familial homes. It was also Nuevo Futuro, with its fighting women on the frontlines, who battled to create *therapeutic homes* capable of taking in and caring for the youngest patients with the most severe symptomatology that threatened

DOI: 10.4324/9781003261490-1

the stability of the organization's foster homes. That was how *Project Sirio* came into being—from *Sirius*, the star that shines the brightest—to care for and treat children and adolescents who presented with serious mental disorders and who were in need of individualized mid- to long-term residential treatment. Today, with over 20 years under our belt, and more than a hundred children treated, our experience in the treatment of these types of disorders is extensive.

1.1.2 On depressed babies

In recent years, developmental psychopathology—historically situated as a development of psychoanalytic object relations theory—has also illuminated and continues to shed the most intense light on this type of disorder.

Back in 1945, Rene Spitz was already describing anaclitic depression in hospitalized babies who were separated from their mothers after the terrible human losses and family ruptures after World War II. They exhibited somatic symptomatology (decline in the developmental quotient, weight loss) and psychic symptomatology (marked irritability, asthenia, apathy, sadness, and weeping, they stopped crying and refused food, withdrew, and were indifferent to stimuli), which could even lead to their death. Both Spitz's observations of "hospitalism" (1945) and Anna Freud & Dorothy Burlingham's (1973) *Reports on the Hampstead Nurseries 1939–1945*, during wartime, proved that babies deprived of a maternal presence and stimulation, suffered severe symptomatology and sequelae. John Bowlby (1979) then focused on the primary relationship between the human infant and its mother, and his seminal theory on attachment has become foundational for all subsequent theorizing on the socio-emotional development of the human subject.

The different types of *bonds* or *anomalous attachment* styles of the baby with its mother or available primary caregiver were studied, and different criteria were established for formal diagnoses. The American Psychiatric Association (DSM-III, 1980) and the World Health Organization (ICD-10, 1992) introduced them into their respective diagnostic classifications for illnesses and mental disorders for children, and criteria have been slightly modified over time. And although the diagnoses are rarely considered to be the most important factor in our clinical understanding, other than in long-term institutional settings, perhaps, attachment theory seems to be receiving as much attention as ever from clinicians and the scientific community over the past few decades.

1.1.3 Learning to be human

The learning of interactional patterns, of human relatedness, starts to take place through the mother, from the very first stages of life. The baby automatically and attentively observes the mother's face, voice, state of tension, of calmness, and ideally receives in return—in a predominantly *mirroring* relationship (Winnicott, 1967)—a response that progressively melds and coordinates itself with that of the child. The mother does not «teach» the child in a sense we could term pedagogical, but rather lives and shows how to live, by processing the emotional states she intuits in the infant. That is when the wonderfully *unique and distinct* tale of *intersubjectivity* begins to unfold, full of intuitions and reciprocating perceptions about what «the other» feels, enjoys, needs or wishes, through the non-verbal communication, the tenderness, and the gentleness in the relationship.

Because for the human subject, as Buber (1958) would have said, there is no *I* without a *Thou*, or in the words of Winnicott (1960), "there is no such thing as an infant, meaning, of course, that whenever one finds and infant, one finds maternal care, and without maternal care one would find no infant". The exchange begins there, in that dialogical movement between two different worlds that overlap and lay the empathic foundations for two people to get to know one another. But in this primary human relationship, the balance of forces is greatly uneven. Hence, the mother's role has enormous power and responsibility. If the mother is lacking the necessary supports, or if she is ill or not up to the measure of this relationship, the child's subsequent mental health could be compromised and it could lead to significant deficits in the construction of the child's personal identity. How might we provide adequate support for these priceless, crucial, primary, and earliest experiences within the mother–child dyad to unfold as unharmed as possible, in our complex and ambivalent affluent society?

The *good-enough mother* (Winnicott, 1971) is attentive, available, adequately perceives, intuits, and responds to the infant's needs;

provides adequate stimuli—through touch, gaze, words, food, serenity, reliability, and tenderness—and sufficient comfort; she is present and available, but does not overprotect; she is able to filter the disharmonic or inadequate stimuli, for the balanced, congruent, and harmonious development of her child ... Can she be found, cared for, and supported in the world of today?

1.1.4 Creating mind in the baby ...

Those parents who have the resources and capacity to consider the baby as a subject, with a mind of its own, will be better able to provide more attuned and adequate parental care—which in the beginning are necessarily intuitive responses to the signals issued by the infant—better parental reflective functioning, and better empathic understanding of the child (Fonagy et al., 2002).

The mother creates a *basic trust* (Erikson, 1963) necessary for developing the pillars of mental health of the human individual. With this *basic trust*, the baby can continue the initial phases of its development and evolution, from its theoretically idyllic and protected state in the maternal womb to an adequately balanced state outside of it, free from the constant lurking dangers that the outside, that life, may have in store. The trusting child who has faith, who is not excessively afraid, who has a secure connection with his/her primary caretakers, will grow and learn, will feel better able to explore, and will be further enriched by the social interactions and environmental stimuli. His/her autonomy and subsequent freedom will, thus, gradually increase in the process with *manageable* conflict. The infant's relationships and early learning will be the pillars and the motor for all other subsequent ones as he or she develops.

1.1.5 ... or generating pathology

On the flipside, *attachment disorder*, a disorder originating in the lack of that necessary *secure base* for a healthy psyche, results in disturbed social relations along with a host of diverse and extensive dysfunctions.

According to the current international psychiatric classifications in use today, DSM-V and ICD-10, two variations of this diagnosis are considered here. These are reactive attachment disorder (RAD) and disinhibited social engagement disorder (DSED) in DSM-V (previously referred to as disinhibited attachment disorder in both ICD-10 & DSM-IV-TR), and they include a long list of symptoms: a disturbance is evident before the age of five; social relations are notoriously contradictory or ambivalent; emotional disturbances are manifested by sadness, lack of emotional responsiveness to others, withdrawal, aggression when faced with their own or another's discomfort or fearful hypervigilance; fragile attachments (ranging from immediate intense attachment to detachment) are a persistent characteristic in their social relationships, with a relative failure to establish selective social relationships, manifested by a tendency to seek comfort in others when faced with one's own distress, the absence of a normal selectiveness in which people to seek comfort, and poorly modulated social interactions with strangers.

Our clinical research has suggested that this disorder can be thought of as a pre-delusional state that is a precursor to paranoia (Herrero, 2009).

Beyond the manuals and the theories, what do we know from our child and adolescent mental health team about the disorders that our children suffer from?

We can now establish that the causes that generate *attachment disorder* are many. In addition to those conventionally recognized as parental illness (maternal depression, psychosis, drug addiction, hospitalization, or prolonged separation from parental figures during the beginning stages of life) and obvious neglect, abuse, and maltreatment, maternal absence due to difficulties in work-life balance in the stressful world of today, or frequently changing caregivers may also contribute to the genesis of this disorder.

1.1.6 On the genesis of empathy

New theoretical developments, supported by recent research in neuroscience, place *the development of moral conscience in the very early stages of life*, with the emphasis on the intuitive, implicit, and emotional aspects of moral behavior, as opposed to those rational aspects, which have figured prominently in decades past (Kohlberg, 1981). Neuroscientific research shows that affect *reciprocity and empathy* are key factors in the process. Evidence suggests that both emotional processes are grounded in our adaptive evolution, that they exist across different cultures, and that they occur intuitively and automatically in social situations rather than being part of a rational and deliberative process. Authors such as Papousek (1981) or Bornstein & Sigman (1986) agree that the most important aspect of moral conscience develops very early on out of the interaction between infants and primary caretakers, and is found in many non-human primates (de Waal, 2006). The universality of *turn-taking* behaviors between mothers and babies across cultures is surprising. «Do unto others what you would like others to do unto you».

Empathy and concern with the Other's well-being, considered a crucial aspect of morality, can be detected as early as the second year of the life of the child (Emde et al., 1991). Thus, when the child is confronted with the stress or distress of the other, he/she not only shows signs of stress or distress too, but also develops helping, caregiving, or comforting behaviors, directed towards the one who suffers. It is also possible to observe distress in the child that is produced by a violation of the standards of behavior, which have already been internalized in the second year. At a very early stage the basic motivational forces for cognitive assimilation—exploring the environment, detecting what is new, transforming it into something familiar—have consequences over internalized norms and expectations, about what is right in the world or is expected to be so. This is the way early standards become internalized. When the child, during the third and fourth year of life, develops narrative capacities, another element in moral development appears: the construction and transmission of narratives to the primary caregivers; allowing for the child to articulate, envision, and create alternatives, something that will be vital in his/her moral development. If one cannot imagine possible alternatives to his/her actions, his/her moral decisions will be limited. For this reason, early development of the child's imaginative capabilities should be considered to be yet another fundamental, necessary and key aspect of early moral development.

1.1.7 Mental health is much more complex than was thought before

These early competencies are now considered part of childhood mental health. They can only be established in a healthy development when the dyadic relationship between mother and baby involves the experience of intimacy through a sensitive and sufficiently available maternal presence, characterized by adequate responses to the infant's needs and the elaboration of implicit mutual expectations. Children who have grown up in conditions of (emotional and socioeconomic) stress and are deprived of nurturance and soothing from their primary caretakers are much more likely to suffer from deficits in this area, especially (but not only) those children who have been maltreated and/or display disorganized attachment behaviors early on (Bernier & Meins, 2008; Carlson et al., 1989; Cyr et al., 2010; Gedaly & Leerkes, 2016; Sroufe, 2005).

In addition, what we know today is that those individuals who grow up under these conditions have a greater risk of suffering from problems later on in life (Carlson, 1998; Lyons-Ruth, 2003; Lyons-Ruth & Jacobvitz, 2016), which include not only dropping out of school, but also teenage pregnancy, and many health problems (Felitti et al., 1998), and also problems in moral development. However, and even though it still seems to come as a surprise to many today, research shows that the long-term prognosis for *early interventions in children with these types of deficits, offers positive outcomes in their behavior as adults.* And the fact is that interventions performed during early infancy, not only result in fewer teenage pregnancies and fewer school dropouts, but also in less delinquency and fewer crimes in young adulthood.

Social analysis of costs/benefits performed by economists (Karoly et al., 2005; Trefler, 2009), not just by educators or clinicians, has underlined the *benefits of investment in early intervention programs in childhood* that prevent the development of disruptive and antisocial behavior, and of serious, subsequent and sustained economic and social costs for society as a whole.

1.1.8 How we address the phenomenon of attachment disorder

The ultimate goal of our work laid forth here is threefold:

- To offer psychotherapy to address serious psychopathology. It is an important part of a tailored, complex, and multifactorial treatment and accompaniment. Referred to as tertiary in medicine, this treatment is nonetheless essential for subjects who already present pathologies that are established, set, and chronic.

- To educate with narratives such as the one offered here, sharing our knowledge and clinical experience with other teams who work in child and adolescent mental health, so that we may disseminate and advance the knowledge we have acquired about these pathologies along with the potential that necessary treatment provides.
- To offer families and professionals interested in the world of infancy, and society as a whole, an essential topic for shared reflection: on necessary policies to care for mothers and pregnancy; on the care of children during the first two years; on the reconciliation of work and family life; on the needed support and guidance for families, including adoptive families; on a more extensive understanding of the etiopathogenesis of very serious and persistent psychic and social problems in adolescents and young adults; on policies for preventive programs to avert mental pathology; and on adequate investments in mental health.

Chapter 2

Therapeutic accompaniment

On a Friday quite some time ago, our team's psychiatrist, psychotherapist, and director asked me what I might consider the essence of my work accompanying the main character of this story. It was during one of our preliminary morning meetings—book-meetings we called them—to decide on how to organize this book. It was the beginning.

Long days followed with my wondering what an *essence* was all about and how to describe one, or if it were altogether possible ... I thought of the word and its meaning, of what the essential aspects might be. I remembered the smell of parks, of the streets we worked on, of the dark corners and those filled with light, of the faint fragrances of my memories, and I began to write.

From diffuse and vivid memories, smells, sensations, and subtle fragrances returned, to lose themselves in the breeze of the days as I wrote. I thought of it like this, because our team's director had invited me to lose myself in my reveries. In all this imagining, accompanied by a trove of papers and notes from our work, in this studying, thinking, organizing, remembering, attempting to extract what was essential in all of them for the writing of this manuscript, lay the elixir. For imagination is where parts of reality and fantasy meet. And what are smells written down on paper, if not *essences* captured in the motley metaphor of language, arising as a means of weaving a thread through the reverie of our recollections! They transport us to the veiled realm of imagination in which we can all share parts of the experience. Perhaps that is what I am now attempting to do.

DOI: 10.4324/9781003261490-2

Throughout these pages, I would like to share my lived experience of what was essential in the process. And what a task! Because I am invisible in it! Those who read this cannot experience my experience, that is only mine. Just as I cannot have that of others, because the experiencing of our experience is that which makes us invisible to the other and lies within us, though it permeates the space between us (Laing, 1968). What a project this was turning out to be then! To launch oneself into making the invisible visible, and the intangible tangible.

I feel still today, and very much so, an apprentice. I have always felt like an apprentice, although perhaps after these long, shared and profound experiences, I might say I feel like a *magician*. But nothing would stray further from the truth, for I was solely a companion. Perhaps with my words, now reflected upon and written, I may conjure up the magic that will allow for the real girl whom I accompanied for over two years, through the long voyage of her life, to emerge and be seen in these pages. Perhaps it is also in this attempt to write, flooded by my own uncertainties as I face the task, where the essential aspects of my work may begin to surface. Maybe even my own experience may actually allow me to convey the process. The elixir of accompanying did not lie in being beside our girl but was perhaps in that carefully constructed invisible space (of alchemy) between us.

The essence of my accompanying resided, therefore, in a creative and invisible space, meditated on, studied, worked-on and alive, where a profound connection was born, which transported Yao Lu to a safe, cared-for and treasured place in which to grow. These pages are an attempt to reflect on the work that took place, as much as they are an invitation to the reader to become a companion on that voyage through the writer's subjective experience of the *construction of a reparative attachment,* with Yao Lu, a little star who risked fading-out altogether.

2.1 Light in the darkness of despair

I met Yao Lu, after having spent the previous year working as a child and adolescent Play Development Coordinator in a marginalized neighborhood on the outskirts of Dublin. My work there focused on enhancing adult attunement to children's needs in parent-child and staff-child relationships in underserved community playgrounds. Before that, I had spent some time working as an educator in our Therapeutic Community in Madrid, which treats children and adolescents with serious mental health problems. These children are also under some measure of protection, due to previous situations of neglect or family vulnerability. I was excited at the possibility of being a part of the team in Madrid again.

Every break of day, in the Irish capital, I would come across a few burnt cars on the streets and landscaped areas where a specter of colorful crystals, sharp slivers of multicolored glass, poked out as the new day's light shone on them. They emerged and peered out from the grass and asphalt, as a reminder of the prickly spines and sharp edges of the lives of the children in that neighborhood. Adolescents broke into cars to drive them to ruin and later give them a grand finale in flames. The next day only steel skeletons were left beside the tears of molten glass on the ground. Amid all this chaos there were children, many boys and girls, playing and exploring the bits and pieces of burnt garbage bags, or climbing up on the improvised jungle-gyms and skeletal remains of the cars recently gone up in flames. Albeit usual, the sight of girl-mothers was no less dramatic. In their most tender adolescence, they pushed their babies around in strollers with their own 30-year-old mothers at their side. Their independence was made even harder still, because before they had established the necessary autonomy, maternity compelled them into regression and increased dependence on their own mothers. Maternity was paradoxically infantilizing.

Playgrounds were locked up at dusk, under the custody of long spiked steel fences that refused to give in to the constant threat of glass, cans, and syringes. As if a part of Diego de Velazquez's painting *The Surrender of Breda*[1], they rose imperiously and sinuously towards the sky in a desperate cry, reluctant to surrender to the desperation and perpetual anguish of the forthcoming days.

And in that scene, as now in the case of Yao Lu, the essential goal consisted in turning on the light at the end of the long dark tunnel of despair so, as in the painting, she could be kept from collapsing under the misfortune of her predicament, so she could, on the contrary, rise and courageously take on the responsibility of a life free from humiliation and move forward.

But go where? Yao Lu had gotten pregnant. We had to call out for *Hope*, or create her. But who was she, exactly? What was she? And most important of all, where could we find her?

Hope was a projection towards a place both far away and near, the possibility of growing somewhere better, of living different experiences, of not being absorbed and consumed by darkness, of legitimating and giving value to the quest for the meaning of life and to fight for oneself. It is in the struggle for the profound value of life, where we, educators, must accompany, inspire, and deeply care for these children and adolescents. It is in this struggle where those who have suffered the vicissitudes of injustice on their own flesh can reconstruct themselves and grow in the face of their painful and suffocating destiny that is closing in on them. Hope is light, the brightest and most fragile of them all, so fragile we should never let it be put out.

Note

1 On display at the Prado Museum, in Madrid, Spain. The painting shows a moment where the Spanish general Ambrosio de Spinola keeps the defeated from kneeling, to respect him and honor him as a near-equal instead.

Chapter 3

The budding bond

3.1 The construction of an attachment; defining the relationship

3.1.1 Being and becoming: survival, transition, and reattachment

I remember when we first met in Madrid. Together with my program director, we met her at the new place where she had been transferred from our Home—our team had already been working with her for over a year—since she had gotten pregnant and had her mind made up to go through with the pregnancy. Though Yao Lu would temporarily live in a maternity home for young mothers, our therapeutic team would continue working with her. On my way over there, I remember thinking how I would approach her, how she might be feeling. In a very short span, her life had been significantly overturned. She had moved and she was pregnant.

I met the gaze of a petite and fearful girl, withdrawn in the airtight bubble of her inner world, the place into which I was to find my way. At least that is how I envisioned her when I saw her, sitting on a small couch, looking at me distantly, protected under the blanket of her folded arms, frightened and apprehensive in her faraway *wordless world.*

Uncertain and overwhelmed by the complexity I foresaw, I peppered her with questions, unsuccessfully attempting to open routes to verbal communication. I was a stranger to her! And in a certain sense so was this type of work for me. The more I asked, the more she withdrew and distanced herself, as if there were an insurmountable space between us. She only responded with small non-verbal gestures, nodding and shaking her head, until … nothing at all.

DOI: 10.4324/9781003261490-3

I reminded myself of my main task: that she could come out of her introverted bubble, communicate and speak. But for that to take place, there needed to be a relationship of trust! I did not know her! Patience ... How stressful! And what a contradiction! Was I perhaps more nervous than she? My anxiety was growing. I did not know how to face her ... *Patience*. And maybe this was essential to our work, because without it all is uproar, tension, urgency, and noise, the subtleties of the hidden world of emotions would remain trapped beneath. All in due time, things would come around, I thought, and left. We could meet again the following day.

The second day, I set off to meet her on my own, without my director. Yao Lu was not available and I was taken by fear. I imagined that her new life circumstances might be closing in on her faster than I had thought, but I needed to be patient. It was essential. And I started making use of what I had (my gift) around the premises: *time*. I walked around the outside of her maternity home. My guess was that she might take a look out of her window, and perhaps seeing me was more reassuring than not. Shortly after, down she came, wearing pajamas! She was reluctant to be in my company, refusing to engage with a clearly spoken «No». So, as something natural to this job, I *prudently* and calmly readjusted. I looked to reconnect, but first with myself. How did I feel? How would I feel if I were she? In an attempt to transcend my small invasion of superfluous words, I shared that I was actually very shy and that, paradoxically, in other contexts, I did not tend to speak much. She seemed skeptical. My anxiety was spilling over and made our meeting more difficult. I was scared that I might be incompetent. Our gridlocked silence also unnerved me. And the fear must have been mutual. I was afraid of being quiet and exposing myself to a space with Yao Lu, and perhaps my silent presence made her uncomfortable, because it exposed her to the silence too. After all, we were nothing but two utter strangers. W.R. Bion (1990) pointed this out as a key dynamic in one of his conferences in his Brazilian Lectures. And was he right! We were both shrouded by a relation of fears we wished to avoid. Simply said, we were just two people, more similar than otherwise (Sullivan, 1953), and our fears, though from different sources, ceased to be anything but normal.

Given the fruitlessness of my words in the face of her non-responsiveness, I directed them to myself as I reflected out loud on my emotions. This was an attempt to cautiously bridge the gap, by acknowledging it and differentiating my feelings from hers. She arched her eyebrows, since in my nervousness my tendency was to talk a lot (and my friends in adolescence teased me for being the silent type!). I tried to wedge my way in through the crack offered by the raising of her eyebrows. It seemed to suggest that I put on the brakes, yet at the same time seemed to point out the need for further clarification. I guessed out loud what her feelings may have been and how I might have felt if I were the one who was expecting the visit of a (known) stranger. «I would also look out the window and hide right back under the covers!». And as I mimicked hiding under them, Yao Lu's laughter emerged, casting a ray of light into the abstruse dynamics of our budding relationship. I slightly exaggerated the mimicry, she laughed yet again, a chuckle surfaced, we laughed together—and something new began.[1]

How is one to lend a helping hand that reaches into a defended and elusive inner world? This was my dilemma: anxiety and uncertainty interfered, and yet I should not be imposing my emotions on her. My emotions were not hers. Instead, *it was important to be ...* to simply *be*, without intruding, much like a mother molding and adapting to the needs of her newborn, intuitively reading and interpreting the child's states. She must be soothing when the child faces the anxiety of a new environment, and not intrude with her own anxiety. Between Yao Lu and me the rest would in time develop slowly, guided by my intuition and empathy. Through the incremental steps of our work, defined by my profound respect for her rhythm, and protected from my own anxiety, a healing relationship would unfold.

Needless to say, Yao Lu was not a baby, nor did I treat her like one, yet she was already carrying a baby of her own. It was difficult, but I was soon able to sense that those were the tentative beginnings of a therapeutic relationship. It was initially precarious and fragile, yet at the same time potentially strong due to the supports of her new situation, which included my willingness to engage her, to meet her, and the many supports that our entire team was about to provide. Yao Lu was quite a little storm of ambivalence during the first few weeks of my work. I can, and will, speak to that!

3.1.2 Notes on Bion, Miller, Winnicott, and others

How to foster a reparative attachment? What do mothers do with their babies? I was surely not her mother, but maybe I could do something similar to what mothers do. A bond of accompaniment, albeit weak and diffuse, had just been established. Yao Lu needed the care a baby might need in order to endure and survive in the wide world of Madrid and to reduce its many risks. What would my accompaniment be like then? Much like the good enough mother's presence: intuitive, adaptive, calm, and containing.

In order for my work to succeed, accompaniment had to focus on «being,» not «becoming». First, that meant trying to understand her and getting to know her. I had to adapt to and try to respond to Yao Lu's affective, emotional, and basic needs, similar to how security and connection are constructed in maternal relationships, as described by D.W. Winnicott (1971, 1975), but from my professional position. It was an exercise of constant reading and intuiting, because although Yao Lu knew how to speak to communicate, she didn't do so very much. She communicated through silence and through her behavior![2]

Just as if I were with an infant, I nurtured the relationship; and through that relationship nurtured Yao Lu. I was there for her if she needed it, as much as possible, even though I was limited to my work hours (four hours a day, three times a week). I always remained attentive and receptive to her negative states of mind, to her anxieties, hopefully in a regulating interaction, that affected and encompassed us both (Beebe & Lachman, 1998). Although I initially had a hard time admitting it, Yao Lu's anxieties also had an effect on me. Back then, I took cover in an observant therapeutic posture, somewhat removed from what was happening to me internally. This allowed me to manage those anxious resonances in which we found ourselves, as we moved— at first without being aware of it—towards generating our "space of thirdness" (Benjamin, 2004, 2009)[3], with the progressive dissolving of my fears and the construction of common ground.

There were times she expressed those anxieties towards me in the form of contempt, rejection, or anger, although they had little to do with me directly. They had to do with her prior experiences with other men; experiences she was not yet ready to tell me about, or perhaps even understand. It was akin to the malaise or discomfort a baby shows the mother when faced with disturbing negative environmental stimuli that produce unrest, although it is not the mother who generates them, but it is she who should learn to interpret her baby's communication, which is not yet verbal. By doing so, and after the necessary and developmentally adaptive fusion of the mother to safeguard the physical and emotional wellbeing of her baby, the latter may develop a new consciousness of self.[4]

Yao Lu was like a little girl, though lacking the basic trust in the reparative relationship we wanted to build. Unable to speak to me of her world in words, she was prey to unpredictable swings that went from angry and tearful outbursts, to diffuse restlessness, and to states of calmness, all of which I had to learn how to read and understand. Our communication was not fluid, as might be easily intuited, but we would work on it.

Obviously, I could not be her mother, despite my mothering attitude. I had sideburns, which a day without shaving would accentuate. I had to patiently build the relationship, without applying pressure, or it would break. I was the new person in her world, and she was also the new one in mine, one whose type of world I had never worked in before, and I had to remain aware of the imbalance my presence could cause.

So there I remained, taking care of the relationship amidst its early thunderous clashes and, through the relationship, I took care of her. Much like a weeping willow, I did not return the anger of her stormy outbursts, and when faced with the jolting winds, I did not topple over but, rather, gently gathered her up between the branches of my containment and prudence, allowing the wrathful wind to slide between them, slowly bringing her back in the to and fro of my soothing position. Bion (1990) viewed this *"capacity for maternal reverie"* as necessary for the growth and psychic maturation of the child or baby. The infant cannot metabolize the anxieties and bodily distress triggered by the external world because it still lacks a fully mature psychic apparatus. Anxieties, pains, and anger are projected onto the mother (or maternal figure), who collects them, digests, and detoxifies them, since she *does* have the capacity (ideally) to modulate those primary sensory experiences, and she can then return them transformed to her infant. A mother with the *capacity for maternal reverie* will hence give back calmness and containment by attending to the possible and by frustrating the impossible. In doing so, the baby—in this case Yao Lu—could gradually receive those harmful elements of her anger and her projected states in a filtered version, and gradually integrate them into her mind.

I found myself in a constant to and fro, very similar to the comings and goings of a new mother who closely tends and gives space to her newborn child on the basis of what she senses is needed. I would survive her rejections serenely. She could destroy me in her fantasy and I would continue to be there for her (Winnicott, 1971).[5] I would allow her to express her anxieties or frustrations, without having to coerce them into satisfying my own narcissistic needs as a helper (Miller, 1981).[6] Otherwise, we would be constructing an «as if» relationship full of smiles, and dominated by false selves (Winnicott, 1965).

Perfect psychic containment did not exist, or at least how to accomplish that was beyond me. All I could do was try to hold her in her angry outbursts, to filter them with what soothing and containing words I had, and hope that she would return to a calm that would allow her to think. This laid the foundation for accompaniment: moments of meeting, others of failure, ruptures, and repairs (Beebe & Lachman, 1996) along a path of increasingly successful affect regulation. By not being reactive to her emotional outbursts, our relationship offered the possibility of slowly disentangling her from the constricting blame that riddled her world with guilt (Barudy & Dantagnan, 2005). But for this we would have to talk, and talk a lot, and for that she was not yet ready.

Our initial conversation seemed superficial. It did not focus on her emotional needs, but on the more mundane ones, such as items from the supermarket she liked, or educational materials I could provide. I needed to see to understand, to listen with my eyes and my emotions to be a true companion. It was crucial to allow myself to feel her experience in a tempered way, filtering it through the glimpses and echoes of my own (Boston Change Process Study Group, 2018; Grossmark, 2016). I had to facilitate the connection, through the great challenges due to her life history. Yao Lu had been a victim of severe physical and sexual abuse. The building of trust was to take place one droplet at a time, with the gradual deconstruction of her mistrust of men, to thus be able to bond with me. Because the springboard for reparation was a world stirring with ghosts and fears (Vaillant, 2004), these fears were bound to reemerge in her relationship with me.

In that affective desert of a tortured world, visited by anxieties and terrors, we cultivated the space and time for our relationship (Vaillant, 2004). The task was a complex and difficult one, of collecting fertile droplets that fell into a world of fears, anxieties, and pains, and that could also revive old hurts that lead to a storm. Yet these storms held the texture of a hidden emotional world, negatively charged as it was by a life history riddled with sexual abuse and maltreatment by men.

As a man, I had to be approached with great ambivalence. In turn I had to be extremely delicate, meticulous, and clear in the therapeutic relationship I wished for us to build together. We had to gradually shape our relationship into a space for positive experiences, so Yao Lu could then use it to soothe herself when she needed to. With the intrepidity of hope, perhaps one day, in her future, she could transfer that experience to her interactions with other men. As a compass in her becoming, she might depend on a transitional object, like a child would count on a stuffed animal or a favorite blanket in an anxious situation so as to self-soothe and recover calm. I would not abandon her after her angry outbursts, nor her risky behaviors. She would not lose that space in which to speak if she so wished. I would work to keep that door open, to welcome her whenever she was ready, receptive to her problematic behaviors as communicative, and hopefully transform them into constructive conversations.

If I was unable to accept those anxieties, emanating either from her or our relationship, how could I ask it of her? (It would make me a hypocrite!) To be able to listen without escaping in hasty reprimands, without judgment; to be able to listen and not just hear, to understand and not just answer, were ways of inviting her to process her own anxieties. If I was able to be there, to listen deeply[7] and remain serene in the hurricane of her emotions, maybe she could begin to tolerate them better, to think about them and not act them out in self-destructive, anxiety-ridden flights. It was essential to remain in her crises, to stay beside her, to soothe, in order to eventually help her out of them.

The work was special. Not because of my (developing) skills, but because of Yao Lu and our relationship. I doubt it could be replicated, and providing a replicable blueprint is not the goal of this book. Rather its purpose is *to invite you into our memories and our artisanal workshop, where we offer a creative way of working and accompanying.*

3.1.3 Dynamics, «the dance of implicit meanings», and «with my pajamas on»

During the first few days, the outlines of an invisible *dance of implicit meanings* began to surface between us. It included the rules of the relationship, even without our speaking of them explicitly. An uneasy silence frequently enveloped us, and I would let her know that if she felt it was too much at some point, I could leave and come back the next day; after all, I did not want to make her feel impinged upon or under pressure. I wanted to accompany her, and if one truly wishes to accompany the other in their world, one has to be invited. After all, her experiences were fundamentally invisible to me and it was up to her to share them or not. Whom she made me into could help or hinder. We were at an interesting crossroads. The responsibility was both of ours. Power, of course, lay mainly in my hands, although it was important that she not feel me as coercive, but rather as a sort of «equal-yet-different-other», so she could begin to value herself, to question her constricted views of both herself as a woman as well as of me as a man, and be able to set her own goals, breaking free from her usual submission to men (Sebastián, 2000).

All of this was dancing around in my head as I walked around waiting for her. I only asked that she come down to tell me, if nothing else: «Go away, go away for today». Free of guilt and with a touch of humor, this was an attempt to help make her rejection real, if she so wished, and in doing so legitimize her part in a relationship that aimed to be one of accompaniment and joint reflection, instead of a prescriptive guide to the right choices through the exercise of my power. «Therapeutic educator», I repeated to myself.

I took advantage of this time to think, and I invited her to do the same. In this attempt to allow the seeds of our relationship to sprout, I also needed to give myself space to approach the moments of silence, and to think about the complex task of accompaniment, as will be fleshed out in these pages. There were days when I went home bathed in anxieties and fears. Which were mine? Which were hers?

How could I avoid going back to biting my fingernails? What kind of relationship was I to establish? Would it be best to be directive or not? What approach would allow me to connect with a girl withdrawn under a blanket of passivity, who was emotionally volatile, and who engaged in risky behaviors? I tried not to dwell on it too much, at least not consciously. I simply listened to the feelings within me as I walked around, trying to find some calm, to master the uncertainties that fluttered about me. One day, I found Yao Lu dressed and ready to go out, although she assured me that nevertheless, she was still wearing her pajamas underneath because she was more comfortable.

Could that be a way of holding on to a sense of safety and comfort to cope with the novelty of walking around with me? Perhaps. So I did not make a big deal of it, yet it got my attention. She was coming along, but not quite completely. As soon as we stepped out the door, she made a small confession:

> I don't get along with my mother at all.

Well now! We were making progress! I leaped with joy internally, but I didn't ask any further questions and just let it stand, since I experienced it as a small concession of hers, as a subtle way of accepting my presence and not as a wish to share her entangled family experiences with me so soon. I did not dare run the risk of going into a more perilous conversation, since the relationship of accompaniment was still tender and frail. I had to be cautious and careful, like a mother with her baby, who helps avoid threats, and comforts with her presence. How to help her feel safe otherwise? It was more important to listen than to respond, to understand than to explain. Listening would help open doors, responding might only lead to a closed one. Understanding would help constructively work out the future of multiple possibilities, explaining would impose one that was not genuinely hers.

As soon as we walked out the door, *the dance of implicit meanings* made itself known, one in which we would be immersed for the next few weeks. I invited her to take a walk; she wanted to show me the places around us she already knew, and I felt how she adapted and tried to mold herself to me. I wanted her to guide me freely, but she was following me! A subtle dance was taking place where the observer (me) was being observed, and at the same time I was trying to observe her observing me. Meanwhile, I was trying not to direct the course too much, and allow her to take the lead. Her insecurity, and the pressure to submit to me and avoid exposing herself, became palpable. While she watched my steps, I watched hers. We almost tripped! We arrived at a supermarket as we both read into the subtleties of the other. The dance repeated itself at the entrance. She looked at me somewhat hesitantly and asked if we could go inside, puckering up her brow and nose, not just wondering if we could go in, but also if she could actually ask and express her desire.

This mutual observation would make itself repeatedly evident even much further in our work. For instance, while in a park after a long conversation about her difficult situation, I tried to look at my watch, but she grimaced so intensely I had to bring it up. Yao Lu told me that since I had checked the time, she thought I wanted to leave her. There were so many things to be aware of! She was taking note of me just as much, or more, as I was of her, and her grimace highlighted our mutual influence of each other.

From the very beginning, this teenage mother and I participated in a mutually influencing system. It was essential to understand this and keep it in mind, remaining aware of the subtleties and paradoxes of our communicational labyrinth. In relationships, the influence of each participant on the other is mediated through reciprocal fluctuations not just of actual behaviors but also of internal states (Laing, 1968). Margaret Mead (1968), Von Foerster (1973), and Nathan W. Ackerman (1962) also suggested a similar dialectic, distancing themselves from a unidirectional psychotherapeutic model in their work with families, and believed the observer to be an integral part (a participant) of the system under observation.[8]

I had a sense that the uncertainties Yao Lu felt in her relationship with me were profoundly disconcerting to her, because they made her question a part of her self. I would dare say, her very identity.[9] It must not have been too pleasant a feeling. If she felt too unstable with me she would begin to feel afraid, and what was essential was for her to be able to feel safe and secure, and eventually free. However, this did not mean that nothing good could come out of the uncertainties of our work together. In the encountering of one's fears, one can also come to terms with a hidden part of oneself, and learn from it. It was a difficult predicament, because fear is also paralyzing!

It would have been easy for me to make decisions for her; to direct her, to guide her, to be the educator who knew best and who was going to show her how to do things right. But would she have closed down? Would the accompaniment have been … a therapeutic one? A rigid approach, centered around my beliefs and functions as an educator (in contrast to accompaniment), would not have allowed for safety, and without safety, she would not have shared. And without new experiences, healing is highly unlikely. I would have simply been absorbed in the censorship of her emotional world, unconsciously imposing the yoke of a gender-based social construct that was protective for me. It would have kept me invulnerable, «masculine» and in control; inviting her, maybe unwittingly, to maintain a seductive passivity she knew all too well, and would have protected both of us from the uncertainties of a new relationship (Altman, 2008).[10] Thus, I would have progressively pushed her away further into her passive and submissive, albeit moody, rejection. I had to generate a question in her—perhaps I could not be like the rest of the men of her history—and from that wondering, elicit a wish to forge a new kind of relationship. As she would state in laughter down the road: «Ah, Javier! You always make me wonder!».

To think and to wonder are part of the essence of living, more than just acting or letting oneself be swept along by ignorance in the dark, prisoner of anxieties past. Yao Lu needed to wonder a great deal, to be able to think and take hold of the reins in her life, so as to shape her future. Doubting, and wondering, was the beginning in regaining control of her present, and she would not have gotten there if I had focused my efforts on teaching, for, as a conventional teacher, I would have kept her bound to her crystalized construct of distant and severe men. Yao Lu had to listen to herself feel, think, and wonder about her way of living with herself and with others. To allow this to happen, I had to listen to her first.

My style at the beginning of the accompaniment leaned towards a position of «not-knowing». It was simple. I did not know her! I practically knew nothing about her. Moreover, I wanted to understand *her experience.* Approaching her with the self-satisfied security of an objective theoretical knowledge that only I possessed would have impeded the emergence of her own self-knowledge.

She was the expert in her way of living, however difficult her experiences may have been, and she was the only one who could speak about them with me. I was a mere guest in her world, and as such I was to be respectful, questioning it only through the new relationship she would establish with me. Her experience was primary to any change; and changes would only arrive with the trickling in of new experiences. As psychiatrist R.D Laing (1968) said, we humans are experiential-behavioral systems.

During the weeks that followed, her attitude was quite ambivalent. Some days I would happily go with her to buy something she needed; others, she would come down to tell me she did not want to see me. At times, she was simply nowhere to be found. On one occasion I found her sitting on a bench, staring at the bustling cars and pedestrians on the street, as if she were looking to surrender to the ebb and flow, draining the noise of her mind in the bustle and tide of reverberating movement. I approached her, sat beside her and, without letting out a word, except a calm greeting, took part in the contemplation of that sustained and oscillating sway of cars, thinking that if she had not wanted me to find her, she would not be there. It was a place I was likely to pass by on my way to meet her, as she very well knew. A short time later, after I expressed my happiness at seeing her, I let her know I was going to check out a storefront that had drawn my attention; I needed some space to think about how to proceed with her. The silence had lasted long enough and I was beginning to feel uneasy. I invited her to come with me if she wanted to, but she preferred to stay seated. When I returned she had vanished.

It was my first test. And I did not want to fail! I had already failed enough in school, because I was usually distracted, going down tangents to some subject I was more interested in, sometimes on purpose and other times not so much, remembering experiences with my family on the other side of the world; the joys, the sadness and the difficulties of not seeing them again until the following summer. Separation was an integral part of my life. I would miss my house, my father who could not come with us, my dog who was also a beloved companion, and in his case, soothing in his silence. In the distances of my past, perhaps

I had had similar feelings to those of Yao Lu, in her life woven of distant worlds, yet joined by an empty and impersonal ocean.

Her escape must have been a quick one, a sudden impulse, because it took me less than a minute to cover the few meters to the storefront. I quickly looked for her, here and there, asking around for her. Later on, after a long period of worry, I was about to give up for the day, when we ran into one another as we headed back to the maternity home. She smiled when she saw me, as if she clearly knew she had not acted appropriately. I did not insist, but instead let her know how relieved I was to find her. And it was genuine! I have no doubt she was surprised by my answer, and we both calmly walked back together, while my mind jumped around with joy at finding her. I still did not have the slightest idea what kind of work I was heading towards, but I felt that I was passing the tests she was setting before me.

There was not much else I could do. Just *being* there I was conveying a great deal, for even "silence, inactivity, (and) symptoms are powerful communications. All behavior is communication. To be is to communicate" (Fuentes, 1983).[11] In this sense, I was communicating: whether she was angry at me or not, present or absent, I was there to support and accompany her in her pregnancy. And I began to be able to *be* there for her, in her process of *becoming*, in a new relationship of accompaniment.

Notes

1 A. Slade (2006) referred to this position as a *reflective stance*, in which the parental figures should not limit themselves to see and understand their children in terms of their behavior—in this case silence—but in terms of their possible subjective and internal experiences. In order to do so, however, I was to recognize and own what was mine, to allow for what was hers, calmly forging what would come to be ours.
2 No matter how hard one tries, as communication theorists would say (one cannot *not* send out messages and communicate) her silence was, simply, a non-verbal and alternative way of doing so.
3 Benjamin (2004, 2009) delineates her concept of a space of thirdness as one co-constructed by the relationship of two subjectivities, transcending the complementary duality of "doer-and-done-to" (one is the receiver and the other an agent, as a therapist-patient relationship might be viewed), creating a new space of consonances and inevitable dissonances, but co-created and co-influenced, shared and connected, similar to Winnicott's potential or transitional space.

4 According to Bahrick & Watson (1985)—«Detection of intermodal proprioceptive-visual contingency as potential basis of self-perception in infancy», *Developmental Psychology*, 21, 963–973—up until 3–4 months babies seem to show a preference for perfect contingencies, as would be a fusional relationship with the mother, and then becoming more interested in high yet imperfect contingencies, as are those of an empathically attuned mother or caregiver from then on (Fonagy & Target, 2006).

5 I was not going to abandon her because of her anger at me, and, as D.W. Winnicott (1971) would say, she could destroy the object (my figure in her fantasy), and it would still survive her wrath.

6 A. Miller (1981) wrote about the fusion of the child's needs to those of the mothers' narcissistic ones (in *The drama of the gifted child*) to the point of becoming the mother's caretaker, which creates a distance from his or her own emotions, and hence the splitting off of his or her genuine and particular inner world.

7 The Buddhist monk Nhat Hanh refers to this as *deep listening*: "Compassionate and deep listening means that the other person [...] has a chance to say what they have never had the opportunity or the courage to say, because no one ever listened deeply to them before. At first, their speech may be full of condemnation, bitterness, and blame. If you can, continue to sit there calmly and listen. To listen in this way is to give them a chance to heal their suffering and misperceptions. [...] While listening deeply to the other person, not only do you recognize his wrong perceptions, but you also realize that you, too, have wrong perceptions about yourself and the other person. Later, when both of you are calm and the other person feels more trust and confidence in you, you can slowly and skillfully begin to correct their wrong perceptions. [...] The intention of deep listening and loving speech is to restore communication, because once communication is restored everything is possible, including peace and reconciliation." (p.17). From *Calming the Fearful MInd* (2001) by Thich Nhat Hanh, with permission of Parallax Press.

8 M. Mead (1968) referred to this as the «cybernetics of cybernetics».

9 Yao Lu and I lived in the same city, but came from different worlds. This could result in head-on collisions if I did not keep it in mind. If not, instead of helping her integrate me into her world, I could just as easily be trying to impose mine onto her. P. Berger & T. Luckman (1991) pointed out the influence of the societal on identity construction, as well as the immense difficulty in changing the crystalized constructs embedded in one's daily living. Changes to these crystallized forms of personhood are felt as a disorienting shock. I could only suggest an alternative reality to the one she had with men, I could not impose it on her—for she would reject it— it was she who would have to gradually take it on.

10 Altman (2008) states that the frequent reluctance of male therapists to treat female teenagers is partially due to social constructs around gender, woven together with the disruptive power of an emergent sexuality that is so difficult to manage in adolescence. He suggests that it is precisely the dissociation of feelings and affects arising in the therapist, triggered by the hyper-arousal and sexuality of the teenage world—combined with the patriarchal power dynamics and the

male therapist's reparative fantasies and illusions of invulnerability—that lead some to acting them out in sexual transgressions or, in the case of the fathers, to avoiding closeness in the relationship with their teenage daughters. The relationship with Yao Lu had risks, but I was clear that these could be avoided. Yao Lu could be seductive if she needed to be, and I would have to cope. I would have to remain aware of my reactions, neither withdrawing defensively nor overstepping boundaries.

11 Author's translation of Fuentes (1983). This is based on the *Pragmatics of Human Communication* by Watzlawick et al. (2011), and the axioms of human communication developed within it. According to these authors, there is no such thing as non-behavior, because "one cannot *not* behave" (p.29) in one way or another, and hence all behavior takes on the value of a message and is therefore a means of communicating.

Chapter 4

First trimester's wait: Who are we?

4.1 The guiding-accompanying-generating a wish for treatment-dance

4.1.1 Building trust

Her problems appeared very early on. Yao Lu had a long history with «the boys». She would frequently take off to meet men in precarious flings, lacking reflective judgment of her experience of them. For days at a stretch, I had no one to accompany and she would explain nonchalantly that she had spent her time with some guy she had recently met. I listened and, over time, she began to want to share those stories with me, and would speak of them briefly in lieu of taking flight, fearing a reprimand.

She eventually began to talk to me about a guy who turned out to be a street thug, her new «boyfriend». In a sweet impulsive attempt to increase the trust in my accompaniment, she wanted to introduce him to me. Almost unexpectedly, I found myself walking beside Yao Lu towards the shared apartment where this guy lived. Before I realized what was actually happening, we were both at the very doorstep of another world. She rang the bell. Seconds later a young individual looked out onto the street from the window on the floor above us, and pulled himself back behind the curtains as fast as he had appeared. Somebody wanted to hide. Shortly after, the door in front of us opened, and a different male in his early thirties appeared with a nervous smile, restless, his face weathered from a harsh way of life. He made an attempt to look calm, but failed miserably, nervously moving his legs, one after the other. He shifted his weight from side

DOI: 10.4324/9781003261490-4

to side, stuck his hands in his pockets, pulled them out, surreptitiously looked up and down the street. He could not keep still! Altogether, he seemed just about ready to dive into the moves of a *breakdance* while Yao Lu asked about her new friend. I began to wonder about this man and she introduced me as her «teacher».

I offered my hand and stated my name, Javier. Firm, direct, sure of myself. He jumped to shake my hand so effusively that he overdid it and gave away his fears and anxieties. In circumstances such as these I had to be very cautious. It was necessary to keep calm, remain firm and steady, so as not to aggravate the fears of others, as well as remain acutely aware of my own. These places and situations were potentially volatile and dangerous. It would be best if nobody stepped over their mark. But the primary person who had to keep it together was me!

It was likely they suspected that I was connected to the police in some way. The less they knew about me the better, because their uncertainty could also protect me. I was concerned by their nervousness; an unease that could mean Yao Lu and the baby she carried were in danger. I remained alert. I could also sense her starting to stir, dimly aware of being in a trap she was beginning to recognize. They did not want to see her. Or was it me? Or was it that they did not want to see her if they knew she was accompanied and therefore less vulnerable? I had to be aware of multiple emotions, my own and Yao Lu's, to use them as our insurance policy and guide and not dissociate them. They would serve me well on many occasions, in the dangerous underworld that lay before us.

All of a sudden I found myself at the doorstep of a world, drug trafficking. There was a rapid exchange of phone calls and pressured voices. «He's not here», was the answer, inscrutable, dry, and indecent. Nobody else came down, even though the lights were on upstairs and it was clear a different person had peered out from the window to look.

Yao Lu's face began to morph. She no longer exhibited the naïve and genuine delight of sharing her friendships with me, she did not exude that childlike happiness that made her shine moments before, but was churning in a whirlpool of turbulent feelings and emotions.

We were told once again that the person we were looking for was not there. Their uneasiness spiked with my presence; they did not know where he was, or when he would return. Yao Lu appeared trapped at the doorjamb before it shut. Skeptical, she looked at me, uncertain and ambivalent, amidst the tugging of two worlds and the rekindling of a visceral fear of a new abandonment, hesitant about going in. She said she wanted to wait for him and disappeared after the man.

I was accompanying her, but from outside. It was my rule of thumb. There were inherent risks to both going in as well remaining outside. Yao Lu did not want me to go inside, she had a sense something was not going well because I was there. I could have tried to keep her from entering, but it would have set me up in a battle I was bound to lose. I was not with her every day, and if she decided to go back when I was not there, my position of power that created uncertainties in those people would have been seriously compromised. More importantly, I never knew what could be waiting behind closed doors in a world like that, so I had to temper my nerves. This was the way I had to work in an open environment.

The individual's nervousness was an unconscious message, to which I responded with attentiveness and caution. I felt that once inside the apartment I might not be able to keep tabs on others' anxieties and fears. I had to remain firm, serene, and steady in my accompaniment. The decision had to be hers, for her future lay rooted in it. Nevertheless, Yao Lu stepped inside, and the door shut behind her. I was restless. I contemplated calling the police. Two minutes later, Yao Lu came back out. Apparently, they had switched their story and now said that the man was undocumented, and she was a minor and they did not like to be introduced to new people.

Fears and apprehensions towards an unknown figure had thrown them off. Clearly they did not want any problems. Days later, as I passed by there once more in search of Yao Lu who had again vanished, I was being scrutinized by vigilant stares from a parked car under the darkness of night. These were dangerous places but, even knowing of the risk, I remember being glad I was there, standing resolute in my purpose. I was provoking some worry in that group, something that could be helpful for Yao Lu. They would probably think twice before treating her badly if they knew she was not alone, but accompanied by me—someone who did not buckle under the constant intimidation of that underworld, but who stood firm, where others might have left or not gone at all.

Yao Lu's feverish worry ratcheted up and burst into a small weeping tempest racing down the street. I went after her, leaving the door to that other world behind us. She managed to slow down, and we spoke in the midst of her raging tears. I tried to relieve her of the guilt, so she would not feel she had made a mistake in trying to introduce me to her «boyfriend», quite the opposite. These supportive moments were necessary. Her wish to introduce me had to be validated and framed as something valuable, since she ran the risk of withdrawing due to the abandonment my presence had caused. Her emotional world needed open doors, not new fences.

It was important to reconstruct and build the trust and the legitimacy of her feelings, to be able to open up new channels for sharing. I could not make the mistake of openly criticizing her «friends». That was hers to do. My job was to help her reflect, to listen to her emotions, which was no small feat, and to validate them. I had to try to get her split-off emotional world to grow under tender care, so she would not unconsciously censor herself in a desperate attempt to avoid the angst of abandonment as she threw herself into precarious and risky relationships. It was complicated, but that's the way things were. Trust had to be built from patience and respect for her feelings. And I was not to allow my own anxiety to take over when facing her risky situations.

We eventually managed to bring into question who she believed them to be. They certainly did not have conventional jobs, as we ran into them on the street on a regular basis. It was important that she reach her own conclusions, and not simply take answers that fit my wishes to protect her, but that were her own. By now, the seed of doubt had been planted. I invited her to think if a lot of people went in and out of the house; if it was normal to have people who did not live there to go in and out of a house all the time. Did they seem like friends and stay, or did they go to pick up something and leave soon after? These questions invited her to wonder and think constructively, hopefully pulling the wool from her eyes that had been pulled over them. These people had a furtive and shifty darkness in their eyes. These questions, without the pressure to give them an answer, echoed within her, opening her eyes critically towards her environment, and she could use them when I was not around. Her situation was a high risk; so part of my responsibility was to direct her attention to real dangers she ignored. One day, in an act of great courage, Yao Lu went straight up to an acquaintance and asked about these characters, if they dealt drugs or not. «Yes». And there was light. Our girl would not tolerate lies, and she took a step aside.

Another man then appeared in her life, and we began to explore the differences with the last one. I encouraged her to proceed with caution in this new relationship meeting, but I was especially tactful so as not to come across as judgmental, and impede the growing trust in our relationship.

I ended up having to wait a day or two, to witness how Yao Lu arrived and said goodbye to him a short distance from where I stood. I did not pressure her to introduce me. She became enthusiastic and elated as soon as we met. She had been to the doctor and she now knew the sex of her baby! She apologized and explained that the young man could only meet at the time of our scheduled meetings. She knew she had not been around when she should have. As I listened to her, I thought of the beautiful moment I could have just missed if I had precipitately jumped to reprimand her for making me wait. I would have missed her delight in sharing her baby's gender with me! Might these fleeting moments actually be the important ones? She already knew she had not been where she should have. More importantly, she was genuinely sorry she had not, which is much more profound than just acknowledging it.

We started talking during the little time we had left. That day she told me that this boyfriend was different, and I encouraged her to give me examples so I could understand more clearly what she meant. She said that he walked her back to the maternity home, while the previous one did not, which I had just been a witness to; he made her laugh when she was serious and, through jokes, managed to lift her bad mood. I invited her to continue to get to know him as a friend because, by how she spoke of him, I had the impression that he could be one. She continued, freely and spontaneously, that...

> Before when I met a guy ... Whoa! I went straight to bed with him.

She was forthright, open in the way she spoke of her behaviors and experiences. It was not a crude moment, but a pleasant, almost tender one. She almost seemed to be unburdening herself of a suffocating weight by expressing it that way. I listened, simply listened, as she began to put into words what seemed like her first positive experience with a man. She went on to tell me she had never had such a good time with a guy before; she felt sheltered, taken care of by him, and he seemed interested in her wellbeing. They talked quite a lot, and she pointed this out as an important difference with her past, because with other guys talking was difficult. She always came across the «fresh ones»—making use of her words here—who were only looking to get her into bed. She began to tell me how she would tune herself off, or tone herself down, in her relationships with men before. She was not speaking about it *per se*, but the shutdown she alluded to was a relational dynamic that I intuitively picked up on in the *implicit dance of covert meanings* of our relationship. It was starting to come into focus.

It was as if she were unfolding from within, and from that new vantage point she was able to look back at herself in a different light. I felt like an explorer of her world, along with her. I let her know she was coming across very differently, more communicative and interactive, as I reminded her of our first day when she had spoken almost onomatopoeically; I imitated her minute gestures and folded arms. The breeze of her refreshing laughter picked up and she said:

> The thing is now I have … I trust you more.

And I felt light, hope and strength, sprinkling over our budding relationship.

4.1.2 Self-protecting limits

Yao Lu decided she wanted to let her new boyfriend know of her secret pregnancy, because, as she said herself, it was starting to show. I neither encouraged nor discouraged it: I walked alongside her decision and would remain beside her throughout the oncoming storms. Upon my arrival, the next day, I noticed she was more withdrawn, as if she had retracted within herself, engrossed in her thoughts. Something had happened.

Her sadness was profound and palpable. I found myself in front of a girl who was tough, very tough, but whose eyes welled up with tears, on the verge of becoming a river. Whenever she was about to lose control she withdrew, her face drawn tight, punctuated by coyish smiles that also betrayed her sadness, in an effort to reabsorb the wetness of her eyes. I searched for an opening to those dammed-up tears, looking for a healthier outlet to her hidden cries. Gently acknowledging the sadness I saw, I gave it words. I invited her to remain connected to her emotions, but not in isolation. I noted that what I saw before me was a strong girl, a very strong one, but she had to know that crying was allowed, that it was valid, that it was acceptable, and that I accepted her. She smiled, she endured, she could hardly keep herself together. I felt how my presence, without urging her to speak about anything in particular, was soothing for her. At last, the tears flowed, and flowed. She felt gloomy, afraid, and somehow without really saying so, lonely.

On the next occasion, I could not find Yao Lu. I called her on the phone; she then appeared downstairs, smiling. She seemed different, and she held another mother's baby in her arms, as if she were finding protection and comfort in him. She told me: «Children are my life!». Protected from her anxieties and emotions by the baby in her arms, she was able to tell me that she had confessed her secret to "the guy", his response being that he really missed his ex-girlfriend. Although the tears had disappeared, the sadness had not. Yao Lu had been grievously injured by abandonment very early,[1] and this made it resonate virulently.

During the next few weeks, we set a task for ourselves that was as troubling as it was complex. The recent incidents had made that primary fear of abandonment resurge. The boundaries in our relationship also began to come into play. I had to be even more sensitive in my dealings with her. She was beginning to feel overwhelmed by loneliness; lonely yet surrounded by people! It was a terrifying loneliness, internal, deep, and painful. It was dangerous too.

During my next visit, I remained alert to possible slippages. It started with everything seeming slightly off. I noticed she was happier, eager to go outside, so we headed downtown to the city. Escorted by her subtle laughter, in a seductive coquettish game, she told me with disconcerting smiles some time ago an «old» man had sat down on a bench at her side, to flirt. When she said *old*, did she mean old like me? Hmm ... I would have to keep that in mind. Something in my gut was telling me she was losing her balance, slipping and sliding, in our relationship. I was going to have to clarify and define it carefully so it would not hurt Yao Lu, but I was uncertain as to how, or even if I was interpreting her subtle behavior correctly.

My attention was drawn less by the content of the story as it was by its timing, immersed as she was in the recent experiences of loss. Moreover, her mother was in frail health, and the highly ambivalent relationship was in one of its conflicted periods, and at risk of succumbing to a permanent rift.

When we returned, she preferred to take a short detour, and once again I found myself walking towards the drug dealer's house nearby. I pointed it out to her: «Why are we going this way, Yao Lu?»—at some point we had spoken about it not being a good idea—«Well, so I can get over it, so...». She stopped herself, slightly frozen. I invited her to continue, for her opinion needed to be legitimized. «So he'll see he isn't the only guy that matters to me». My prior faint alarm turned into a full-blown red alert. I tried to wriggle myself out of the mistaken entanglement she seemed to be trying to weave, and I brought her back to the relationship of accompaniment. Gently but clearly, I pointed out and reaffirmed the subtle, yet clear boundaries of our relationship. They were important. They protected her: *remember that I am your educator, your accompanying-educator, not a "friend"*. I could not allow her possible confusion to take hold, so I took great care to point out the boundaries.

Yao Lu's unmet emotional needs, which were the undercurrents to these behaviors, were very likely rooted in the confusion that childhood abuse and maltreatment generate in children. They were a very important aspect of our work. If we were to work towards healing, without opening up new wounds, we would have to listen to the unspoken and contemplate the hidden. The boundaries and limits in our relationship were meant to hold and to protect Yao Lu, but the confrontation of their limits also brought to the fore the part of her that had been injured at the earliest time, and that inevitably reignited that pain. So, while these limits had to firmly yet gently take her back to the relationship of therapeutic accompaniment, I needed to do so without needlessly inflicting a new big injury, while not completely avoiding the resonances of the old either. Yao Lu needed no one to make her feel more hurt, but would it be an inevitable part of the process? (Levin, 1993, p.xiv).[2]

I could have ignored what she was saying, pretended to be unaware of what she was telling me, but it would have been nothing but another way of plunging her right back into confusion. To intervene as I did had the goal of limiting this type of slippage later on, for in our interactive communication, being mindful of what I said had an impact on what could happen next (Watzlawick et al., 2011, p.113). We had to increase clarity in our relationship, so we could build trust and create a sense of security.

To have brought it up too brusquely could have been felt as having the boundary thrown in her face, an aggression from one who was supposed to be taking care of her. Nevertheless, the hurt of her old injuries was reawakened, then and there, and she conveyed the depths of her feelings through her behavior. My asserting the limits of the relationship likely produced the echoes of previous men in her life, who were emotionally distant, rigid, and insensitive. When we reached the maternity home, in lieu of saying goodbye as we used to, she walked on straight inside, fast, her eyes fixed ahead of me. I tried to prevent her from wondering whether this was the end of our relationship by inviting her to think about what she might want to do on my next visit; our meetings would continue. My hope was that in the repeated act of rupture and repair (Benjamin, 2009) within the necessary boundaries of the relationship, all the while acknowledging and legitimizing her feelings, lay the protective elements of a shared and maintained intersubjective space, at least partially. We briefly exchanged a few words and she left. She retreated to her inner world. The fear of abandonment was the deepest feeling and Yao Lu seemed to disintegrate without the support of the self-confirming *other*. At the time, I sensed a mass of barely differentiated feelings in her, and amongst them, notorious and feared, loneliness returned. The boundary and definition of our relationship had been necessary, even at the risk of destabilizing her. I was worried.

She spent the next few days eluding my company, telling me she did not want to talk. She was tired. I was being explicitly excluded, as she tucked herself away into the dark recesses of the Internet, a difficult world in which to accompany her.

Opening windows to an inner world, and the construction of a space for play

It was difficult and unsettling not to know how I would be received each day, whether she would be there waiting for me or whether I would have to go looking for her. I had to constantly exercise patience and self-control to keep my anxieties at bay. I had a feeling she was surrounding herself with a nefarious crowd that she was not yet ready to talk to me about. If I tried to create small talk, Yao Lu let me know. One of these times, she said:

> You talk a lot, like my mother.

I slammed on the brakes, regaining control over my angst. Yao Lu demanded patience. Red flags were going up in all directions. I tried to be less intrusive. With a smile, I responded that we had hardly spoken recently, hoping the humor might open a door. I had to keep it short though, for I would undermine my efforts by explaining it. It would not be too clever of me to try to make her speak either—and I told her so—that was for her to decide. So I gestured and mimicked as if opening her mouth to free hidden words, and she chortled with laughter.

I had to respect her pace, and not give in to my urgency. She did not want lectures, and I was not interested in giving them either. Shortly after, breaking a silence that felt comfortable and seemed to be validating to both of us, she asserted she was going inside, to her room. Had I not allowed it, I would have discredited the recently achieved mutual respect. She went up and I had a chance to think. And think I did.

These were moments of internal crisis for me. I felt expelled, prohibited from being by her side. Hours and days went by, and we barely exchanged a few words. But once we came back together, after a short vacation of mine, I let her know I had been thinking of her and how she was doing. I accompanied her without actually being there, at least in the insight of hindsight, and more and more so in her voyage into the future. All these moments were delicate, important, and required great prudence. As she would let me know later on, she had not wanted to speak at the time because she knew I would not like what she was up to.

She started speaking to me of a new boyfriend, and I invited her to explain the differences compared to the one before. Once she began talking to me about their relationship I found it worrying. Her treating psychiatrist and I did not yet know quite how worrisome though. Yao Lu and her boyfriend did not talk together that much, she felt his control through insistent phone calls, and he wrapped her up in elaborate fantasies of taking charge of her yet-to-be-born son. He was intrusive, subordinating her, and at the same time promising protection, not only for her, but also for her progeny. He threatened to delete her number if she did not speak with him and, ultimately, to abandon her, while on the flipside he proffered the promise of protection. Danger signs. She began telling me about what her relationship with him was like days after they met. She met him on the Internet. We will call him Marcelo.

Something in the way she told me the story was irksome, and sensing that I had to protect her, I trawled the Web with a few usernames and other data Yao Lu shared with me. Not long after, I stumbled upon a worrisome Internet ad she had put up. Our girl's despair was rising.

Days later, after a long while searching for her unsuccessfully, I finally managed to find her. She did not want me there with her, and there seemed to be something gnawing at her from inside. My gut said I was to stay close, and gently encourage her to express her feelings, even if it meant intensifying her momentary crisis. She was at the brink of exploding in rage, yet she was barely open to communication. She was the picture of a girl about to boil over. With sharp monosyllabic responses, she swiftly stomped away. I walked by her side to interpret and translate the emotions I saw, and to reconnect to her feelings. I had to tolerate her behavior. Off we scurried down the street, as I gently tried to open up doors.

Those eyes look sad. And here I was thinking it was anger! I must have been distracted!

I'm sick of everyone!

Of me? Oh man! Well I thought we got along. I must have been so confused and distracted!

Of my mother and my boyfriend! They're a couple of...!!

I took responsibility for my confusion and distraction. Not getting it was a problem of mine, not hers! I also did not react judgmentally. To do so would have triggered a defensive attitude in her. By responding in this way, her resistance dissipated in a constructive exploration of the moment we shared. Yao Lu was about to burst into tears.

You look overwhelmed.

Yea. They're so annoying! I'm going to keep the child and do whatever I want! Besides, my friends at the maternity home are with me on that! I'm sick of this!

Of course, maybe you're needing more respect, and for them to stop telling you what you have to do. You're a 16-year-old girl now and want to make your own decisions.

I'm going to break up with my boyfriend right now!

I was stunned. Hitting the right notes had made her feel understood, and from the understanding she could feel accompanied. Wanting to break up with the guy was coming out of the blue. Putting her feelings into words was very difficult for her, perhaps because doing so involved thinking and reliving the very emotions she was trying to elude. Talking must have been terrifying then! Fear increased her anxiety, and with the increase in anxiety the capacity to find words to describe those emotions shut down. By getting Yao Lu to talk, I was also trying to reduce the risk of impulsive behaviors.

A game suddenly came to me, and we stopped before a bench where we set up a triangle.

i   *The relational triangle*

You need three people for a triangulation to form. Let's imagine, for example, two educators who are part of the same team (the same would apply to parents), but do not think positively of each other, and are unable to address their difficulties. Because of this, they either avoid each other or simply ignore these difficulties. These educators are represented by the letters A and B (Figure 4.1). Both interact with a specific child, represented by the letter C.

Perhaps A does not agree with B's way of working, and believes C needs to be approached differently or needs another type of intervention. Maybe it is the other way around, and B feels that A is undermining all his/her previous work with C.

If both of them work with the same child and are unable to speak openly with one another about these differences, they will consciously or unconsciously avoid meeting each other, or worse, actively undercut each other. If they do not deal with their insecurities by talking about their troublesome relationship, nor make the effort of reflecting on their feelings, it is likely these frustrations will harden their choices to avoid each other. But that does not mean that they cease to communicate, just not directly. Instead, their communication will then get indirectly channeled through C, as they progressively distance themselves from each other. Let's look at an example:

A: Hey C, I don't think you should be playing with your toy model until you've finished your homework, and especially after your behavior a short while ago.

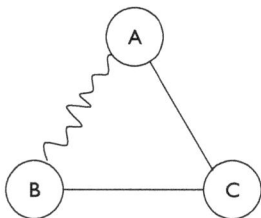

Figure 4.1 Conflict between two adult members (A and B) of the triad is represented by the jagged line. They both seek to have a strong connection and/or relationship with the child (C), represented by a straight line, but are not united in their task of educating together.

C: Well B lets me do it because it calms me down. I'll get back to work in a half hour!

A: Stop playing right now and sit down. It's not the time to be playing and it doesn't matter what B told you. I'll have a word with him/her later on.

[A takes the toy model while C gets upset, angry, and disruptive. A takes off while mumbling in a low voice, that he/she will definitely have a word with B—«B's going to have an earful about this! Here we go again!»—with a discrediting tone towards B].

C: Go for it, when B gets here I'm going to play with the model and you won't be here anymore! [the child quips from the bedroom].

What just happened here? A has become more irritated with C, but in reality his/her anger does not come from the child, but is stemming from the troublesome relationship with B. Their disputes, riddled with their insecurities, overtake the difficult task of educating a child. The differing positions they adopt with C are then made into the primary issue. If A and B do not speak about their difficulties, and if they aren't brave enough to speak about their feelings in a situation such as this, it is likely that, without being aware of the reason, they will begin to find themselves more irritable, unconsciously channeling that frustration through their relationship with the child. And the child will also become more irritable, creating an atmosphere of insecurity for him/her. He/she will no longer know what or whom to follow. Something similar occurs in families.[3]

The following diagram (Figure 4.2) depicts what the triad might look like following the previous quarrel. If the underlying problem is not dealt with and persists, it is possible that the B–C relationship intensifies, but only to the detriment of the necessary overall educational work with C, who needs a strong and consistent A–B dyad.

If the differences between A and B go unaddressed, C would most likely get pulled into a confusing and emotionally dangerous environment, reflecting the conflicting messages of the educators—messages that are more about the disputes between them than about the problems of the child. This is a common occurrence in almost all

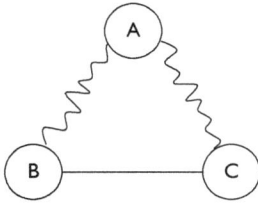

Figure 4.2 Conflict between two adult members (A and B) is not resolved, and it plays out in the relationship between A and the child (C). Meanwhile B and C have entered into a coalition against A, which undermines the overall task of educating/parenting, and the stability of the child's enviroment.

relational contexts! Change the word «educator» for «parent» and we stumble upon a common pattern in many families.

Examples such as these abound:

Father: Tell your mother I will not ... You know what your Mom is like ...

Mother: Your father says he doesn't want this or that. What should I do with him? I can't stand him. Tell him ...

The child absorbs the tensions that have little to do with him/her and often acts out behaviorally. In doing so, the child "acts out" tensions that have not been translated into words since the parents don't speak to each other and attempt to hijack the child in an coalition against the other.

Father and mother speak to each other through the child, since their lines of communication are in a state of disrepair. This "manipulative triangulation" (Linares, 1996) may intensify as the parent's irritability directed towards the child increases. If it happened any other way, they would run the risk of facing each other. Perhaps the child's irritability and disruptiveness might intensify as well! And at that point the parents (or parental figures) will come together to reprimand him/her, so the child becomes an unconscious actor protecting the parents' relationship from falling apart further, as he/she brings the parents together against him/her.

If this takes place frequently, this pattern becomes entrenched, where the parents may end up communicating with one another exclusively through, and against, the child, and the irritability of the triad increases. Unable to speak to each other, the intimacy in their relationship evaporates leaving each isolated and parched. The problem is that this dynamic appears «functional» to the parents by allowing them to avoid the problems in their own relationship—but the child is trapped, holding his/her parents' relationship by a thread, and unable to find his/her own way for him/herself and emotionally separate from the parents.

How might this manifest itself in the child? Paradoxically he/she might show more signs of defiance, or more emotional and behavioral problems, or arguments may increase between the parents/ educators (without the necessary discussions of course), and they might channel their problems into an oppressive preoccupation with the child. Perhaps they might even blame the child—«You make us argue! You are going to make us get divorced!»—attributing to the child a responsibility that does not belong to him/her.

Triangles are to some degree inevitable. Lerner (1989) suggests that they work to manage our anxieties, to keep them at bay. She believes that when a triangulation is undone and people relate to one another directly, without summoning a third, complicated feelings may surface, but it can also provide an opportunity to learn about oneself. (Lerner, 1989, p.170). Simply think of a young man who talks with his friend about the difficult relationship he is in with his girlfriend. «Unloading» his anxieties with a «third», while temporarily helpful, does not put an end to them. That can only be done within the relationship itself.

In my work with Yao Lu, I became part of triangular constellations with third parties whom I did not interact with, her "boyfriends" for instance. I had to be mindful of the anxieties that these others— Marcelo, in this case—evoked in her when they sent her conflicted messages of protection combined with physical and emotional threats and maltreatment, and topped off by overt criticisms and judgments of her. But Yao Lu did not yet feel safe enough to tell me too much about these individuals, and their abuse remained secret.

For these reasons, the team opted to postpone my having regular contact with Yao Lu's mother. The thinking was to temporarily insulate our relationship and to minimize the risk of another intrusive triangulation, for it would likely inhibit the growth of our

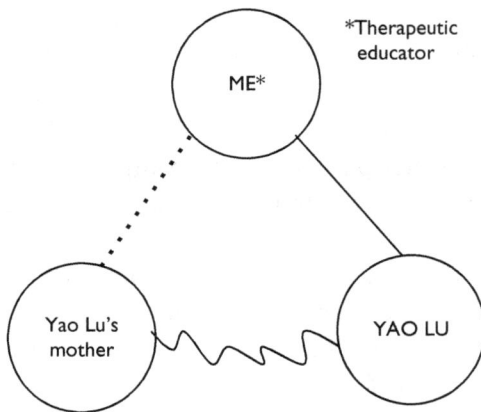

Figure 4.3 The dotted line in the figure represents purposeful distance and a weaker connection between Yao Lu's mother and me, to intentionally enhance my connection with Yao Lu (represented by the solid straight line). This fostered a therapeutic alliance within our relationship. As a result, Yao Lu could speak of the conflicted mother-daughter interactions more freely.

relationship and flood it with anxieties that I would find more difficult to manage (Figure 4.3).

For instance, her mother could try to air her worries with me, and seek me out to help allay her anxieties. Yao Lu could then experience this as a coalition against her, hindering the construction of our bond. On the other hand, I also had to keep the difficult relationship between them in mind, since we wanted to reverse the growing estrangement. Besides, I had plenty of other triangulations to also contend with: Yao Lu's underworld boyfriends; her home for pregnant adolescents, and most importantly, the therapeutic community home. It was decided that family work would take place between mother and daughter with our psychiatrist instead.

Let's now return to the moment when we were walking back to the maternity home. She was marching on, unsettled and angry, practically running as I was trying to give a voice to the emotions written on her face. Her plan was to break up with her boyfriend Marcelo.

ii   *The therapeutic triangulation*

Yao Lu had great difficulty standing up to a man, but she was managing to do so with the help of her anger. We had to take advantage of it, so it could be constructed into a positive experience, not one saturated by pain and anxiety. It was important that she not use her anger to isolate herself and hide, whether inside herself or in the maternity home, where I still had no access. The full-blown crisis offered the opportunity to work on the feelings together. And it had to happen now!

I stopped her, and facing the empty bench, with surprise in my voice, I suggested that we play-act something with that new boyfriend of hers we were both thinking of. She stopped in her tracks. Surprised, with a twinkle of curiosity in her eyes, she took a look at me first, then the bench, and then me again. I invited her to imagine he was sitting there, in front of *us* (*a fortifying us*). Might there be a risk of re-victimizing her by bringing Marcelo into a fictional game with her? Perhaps, but I felt it was minimal, since she had her anger at her disposal. If she could direct it towards the oppressing male figure and stand tall instead of suppressing herself before him, it would be empowering. I was there to support her.

We were in a rehearsal of sorts for her relational life. A kind of *therapeutic triangulation* if you will. Yao Lu, who usually dared not express her feelings and address her abuser, but adapted and submitted to him instead, could use me in a fortifying coalition, directing at him the messages of her split-off voice through me. Thus she could also listen to the echo of her otherwise unexpressed feelings with greater clarity, as she timidly put them into words and I repeated them to amplify their strength (Figure 4.4).

Yao Lu was immersed in triangular relationships, as we all are, but her biggest troubles emerged with Marcelo. She suppressed her feelings in his presence. These were their relational rules, and in their *implicit dance of covert meanings* she subordinated herself to him. In addition, Marcelo, as others had before him, offered the pseudo-security of belonging to him, thus «protecting» her not only from the world out there but also from her own bewildered inner world. Berliner (1958)[4] wrote "masochism does not simply mean to defend against hate, [*be it abandonment or retaliation in Yao Lu's case*] it means to attempt to save love through suffering" (p.46). And it seemed, in essence, that in her submission to men, she was longing to be found, hoping to be recognized in her complexity... Loved, and perhaps after that, she would be able to transform the pain drawing her to the abuser into something

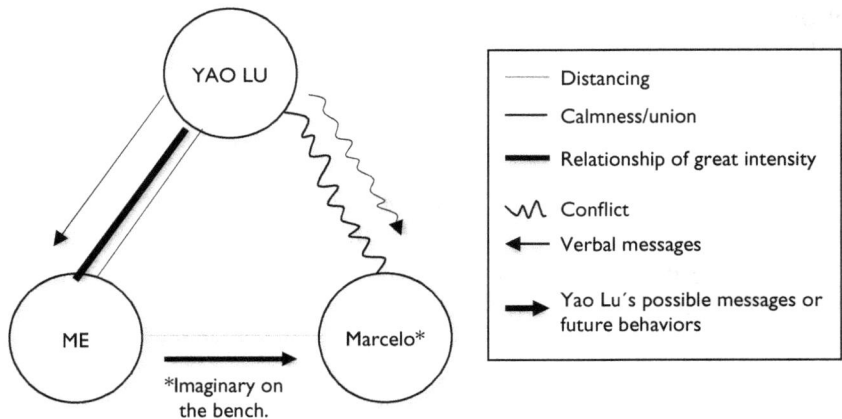

Figure 4.4 Yao Lu told me of her thoughts and feelings about Marcelo (represented by the thin solid arrow). I then playfully directed those comments to him more loudly and confidently (thicker solid arrow). Albeit in play, through this process, she gave voice to the conflicts she usually silenced with him (represented by the jagged line and jagged arrow). Our relationship and alliance strengthened as a result (represented by the solid lines).

different, although the attempt to heal herself this way was futile, as Caflisch describes in a case with a very similar dynamic (2012).

Our girl's submissiveness and her at times masochistic submissions, could be considered a perversion of surrender (Ghent, 1990),[5] rooted in a wish to be seen, understood, known, and hence loved. Handing over her agency to the other—in moments that might be termed dissociative—could be a nebulous, hypnotic, and spellbinding experience for her (Bromberg, 2003), which allowed her to feel "complete"; because in those moments, she could feel "truly" herself,—or at least "one with" an eluded and dissociated part of her identity as an abused girl. In very hidden recesses of her being, she could also feel more whole in the re-encounter with her split-off parts, though this left her at their mercy too (Caflisch, 2012). But what we were aiming to do in our relationship was precisely to salvage those parts, to reclaim the lost feelings, to reintegrate them into a less fragmented way of functioning. Playing them out through "safe surprises" (Bromberg, 2003) in the relationship of accompaniment, perhaps she could literally pull her part-selves together as she surfed the waves of "safety and risk", without being flooded by the tsunami of "affective hyperarousal" (Bromberg, 2008).

In front of the bench, after looking at it curiously, she turned and looked at me again somewhat incredulously:

> I don't know, I don't know...
>
> Wait up, wait up Yao Lu. Look who happens to be there! Well... imagine Marcelo is sitting right here on this bench. Right here! What would you say to him?
>
> Not sure. [Her face changing from hesitation to a timid and curious smile]
>
> Well, if you don't feel brave enough, I can help you... check it out: S'up Marcelo? [and I turned to Yao Lu with an inviting gesture for her to proceed...]
>
> If you want you can whisper it to me and I can let him know on your behalf. Take a look at the guy! He's right there! [I put my ear up close to her and she began].
>
> That he leave me alone. That I'm breaking up with him.

Her soft voice, suppressed in her relationships with men, thus began to make itself heard, a voice that could otherwise only be appreciated intuitively in that subtle *implicit dance* of my first day. I repeated her string of words, directing them in humor to the empty spot on the bench, maintaining a severe tone and creating a protective barrier to bolster her strength against the aggressor. She added «Douchebag! –*Cabrón!*», and we proceeded to slog away, as she yelled out «You're such a pain!» and a very juicy etcetera, and I periodically interjected positive messages directed to her. This triangulated communication of sorts, was an attempt for our girl to be able to say «NO!» in the future, to defend herself and live her life as a whole person, without splitting up to fit into a forceful submission, and instead to find her self in healthy relationships.

It was important for Yao Lu to positively redefine herself before an abuser. My messages were meant to help her grow, to help her face the oppressing figure. This put me in a role akin to an auxiliary ego (Moreno, 1978). Although I spoke in the third person, Yao Lu could take the message, a message she might not have allowed herself to voice. She could look at it, work it over in her mind, and perhaps even make it her own. Most importantly, this was done with the required detachment on my part that gave space to her agency.

> Yao Lu is an intelligent girl, who wants to be respected! Beat it Marcelo! Yao Lu likes to make her own decisions about what she wants to do with her baby, because she thinks a lot and will want to decide what's best! Besides, if she decides to give him up for adoption or keep him, she'll be the one deciding. She doesn't need you to boss her around or organize her...
>
> Yao Lu doesn't need you to control her. Yao Lu is a smart, strong girl, who takes care of herself and likes to be treated well!

Maybe she could begin to introject this self-image in a nascent narrative of her life, one in which she could stand up to those who wanted her to submit. A dim light flickered, peace began to spread, and her expression gradually turned increasingly serene. In the overlap of our playing fields,[6] we were rescuing her voice that had been silenced by others, and that she had silenced for others. We were playing the *mutual game of accompaniment, we began to share, in new therapeutic space of recognition and meeting,* tailored to her... perhaps to both of us.

A door to trust also opened up, and Yao Lu started to show me an endless list of calls and texts she had saved. They were suffocating. Once we opened the door to that world, she began speaking to me about Marcelo during the days that followed. Her descriptions portrayed him as «brazen» in both his words and his behavior, as invasive and oppressing in the realm of sex. It was difficult to get a clear sense of how she felt with him, because she tended to block off her painful experiences and these only seemed to flicker faintly in her darkness. Nevertheless, I sensed she did not feel good about the relationship, which she communicated through her irritation and impulsive outbursts directed at me as we talked about it. The complexity of her world included a significant dose of *impenetrability.* Her experiences were covered by a cloak of confusion and mistrust, rooted in her noxious, abusive, and stormy relationships with practically all the men that had been in her life—and I could not extricate myself from that category.

Marcelo ratcheted up the pressure with an avalanche of phone calls and insistent texts. Our girl managed to tell him that the relationship was over, that she was breaking up with him. She said so explicitly, in her own words. She gathered up her courage and stood firm, this despite a downpour of calls. Yao Lu was growing angry. I remained beside her. She looked at me with earnest eyes; he was saying nobody would help her if she left him and, implicitly, that she had to remain subdued to him. But Yao Lu was strong, at least for the moment. He was nobody to say that to her, as she put it. This was a half affirmation, half-question. She had us! Right? I was supportive, she was going through a trying time.

I knew how badly she felt; I understood how lonely and scared she was. And just like the psychoanalytic author Stephen A. Mitchell pointed out, her affective states and emotions had an impact on me, evoking similar states in myself that I had processed (Mitchell, 2010, p.61).[7] Further, as Scott Peck notes, it does not escape children when their parents (and educators) are able to empathize with their pain. Though they may not be overtly grateful, it helps them learn to deal with suffering. (Peck, 1990, pp.104–105).

A few days later, I sensed that she was very tense, and invited her to go shout it out a few times in the park, to let out her bubbling anger in an appropriate place and in a contained, and containing, way. She smiled the second she heard me say this; it did sound almost comical. She felt understood and we swiftly took off for our afternoon walk.

Her feeling of security, and insecurity, in our relationship depended a great deal on my capacity to contain such anxieties so that they would not boil over. If I was unsuccessful, it was important that we both be able to regulate them together as equal-yet-different-others. Ours was a relationship where I had more power, though I frequently tried to refrain from imposing it to make it more likely for her to own her independence from me too. So she was "out with the bad air, in with the good", as she cleaned out some of the hardened anxiety and anger. If I didn't manage to recognize her and "see" her, the toxicity would spread further. The splitting off of her emotional world would increase, and she would either submit herself to me, or withdraw. It was important to break that vicious circle and liberate her from the feeling of impending emotional disaster, which she would describe to me when she felt safer. She was like a baby who lacks a *good enough mother* (Winnicott, 1953), a mother who could help her filter and transform the excess anxiety-inducing stimuli in a soothing space. Instead, without the help of the mother, the baby is compelled to re-absorb his/her own anxiety without it being detoxified, and, in addition, it now also carries the mother's own anxiety. The baby then, in a terrible moment, unable to tolerate his/her own cries, dissociates them, relegating them to a lost and hidden emotional world.

Our girl already presented behaviors we could term *dissociative* (she smiled instead of crying, kept quiet when she might have yelled, gave thanks instead of rebuking and protesting), and my task became to help her connect to the original opposite, or rather to help her *be as she felt*, and with it to feel harbored, thus *reducing the terror of her own emotions*, so they could be expressed. Yao Lu needed to be able to continue digging-up and processing fragmented archaic and chaotic experiences. I had to create a soothing environment to modulate them, to provide a calm listening that would allow for the possibility to think, to accept those contradictory, confusing, out-of-control emotions in the space we shared. In that space, she could let her feelings be free and express them (within certain behavioral limits) without subordinating herself to me. At the same time, I had to be responsible for my own feelings in order for our intersubjective context to allow for her individuality to come to the surface.[8]

The way she began speaking, and the increasing tension in her face, led me to suggest that we find a different place to speak, before she boiled over. Conveying that I was picking up on the ratcheting up of emotions, I suggested that we get out of there. Though I had to resist the urge to firmly shut her down to get her to stop, it was most important that she feel sheltered, contained, and recognized. I legitimized her disgruntled state with the possibility of shouting out a few times, but this shouting should occur in a safer venue than our current surroundings. Yao Lu needed to vent her feelings, but not there. My cue to go to the nearby park set a limit to her tone in the maternity home. An environment with mothers and babies could get loud, but it had to remain as an environment of tranquility. Thus, speaking in *motherese,* my calm words rocked and swayed our girl's anxieties, providing a soothing environment for her to vent her anger safely. The night before, as a result of an argument in which she lost control, they had had to call the police, so our girl was on paranoid alert.

Yao Lu had the forebodings of an unwelcoming future and summed it up in succinct and powerful words that echoed later on in my mind:

> My future looks real bleak.

iii Crafting a story: Metaphors and instruments for thought

Sometime around then I had given our girl a book about a desperate young woman. I presented it to her by reading the beginning out loud. It made reference to the confusing meeting between the world of children and that of adults, a much harsher one, yet the book began as a fairytale. She was fascinated. The time had come to begin building in hope into her story. We also read a short narrative by Jorge Bucay[9] about an elephant that surrendered to the misfortunes it faced from early on in life; and how, fully grown, he remained tied to a small stake in the ground, a hostage to a life he now had the potential to change. There was an implicit and powerful message in the text, «You can change your situation», hopeful rather than bound to the despair of the moment. If there was a will there was a way, and the catastrophe of despair was to no longer want to find a way out of her predicament.

We would read stories about loneliness and estrangement despite being surrounded by others. The powerful messages and metaphors of the tales implicitly invited her to receive the help and support of the accompaniment amidst the moments of despair and crises. There were days when Yao Lu, albeit surrounded by many, felt stranded on a deserted island, powerless. It was a loneliness with a vicious punishment since the worst is to feel lonely even when others might want to be there beside you!

These stories would accompany her during my short absence for a vacation, as a means of keeping me with her. Full of metaphors, they also served as a way for us to get closer to deep internal issues otherwise difficult to get to, by helping her gain words and funnel oxygen to her emotions without having to tackle them head-on.

Thus we were entering a cloistered emotional world, limited by her underdeveloped voice and restricted emotional vocabulary, renovating and rebuilding it in our conversations as we wove in the new experiences of her daily life. Later on, we would speak of thunderous minds and deafening lightning to describe moments of anger, as the use of metaphor provided some protection while amplifying the subtlety of affect. In line with Bruno Bettelheim's ideas, the task was to bring her inner world into order and thus her life more broadly too. Young Yao Lu often felt bewildered, so it was especially important that she was given the opportunity to learn about herself, and make sense of the complex world in which she had to live. The stories helped us do this. Together we safeguarded the hope implicit in the tales, praising it and giving it value so that we could salvage the hope left in her life, and I could help her understand her conflicted feelings (Bettelheim, 2010, p.5).

We were re-reading the first few pages of a novel about a girl who would become a prostitute, and in the midst of questioning its romanticized view, she interrupted me and said:

Javier … Can we speak about something?
Of course.
Well… Hmm … The thing is I'm wondering about telling you something … Well … Hmm … It's just that I put up an ad …

She then began telling me, behind bashful smiles, that she had put up an ad offering herself for money, and that that was the way Marcelo had found her. The novel had begun to stir up and reorganize her way of thinking about her own, without any intrusive inquisitive questions from me. I reassured her and remained non-judgmental as she trembled with anxiety she explained that her ad was up online. She was worried, since he knew where she lived, and she was afraid. When I sensed that she would categorically be on board, I suggested we go to an Internet parlor together and delete it. She was up in a flash, as if she were recharged with new energies, and we were soon walking along the street. She started telling me, in a torrent of words, that there were quite a few things she had not yet told me about. All in due time …

From the very beginning, I did my best to *respect her setting of the pace*, which our director, from the office and her computer, frequently reminded me of, notwithstanding my worried urgency. So even here I refrained from pushing her to speak, taking care not to step out of our relationship of accompaniment and the frame my visits took place in. My accompaniment could not be coercive. It was important that Yao Lu was the one to draw parallels between her life and the fairytales, and act according to what was awoken in her by reading the stories. This therapeutic approach, in the spirit of Bettelheim, allowed her to truly mature, whereas telling her what to do would have replaced her being beholden to her immaturity with her being beholden to me (Bettelheim, 2010, p.45). The decision was hers. Though not true fairytales like Bettelheim's, the stories we read were intentionally loaded with endings full of hope to help her visualize, think and project herself into brighter futures, far from the nightmare of her past that lingered in her present.

After a long while facing the computer, searching for and eventually remembering the passwords, we pulled down her advertisement on the Web. A new day was dawning as she softly sang by my side, enjoying the music videos of the time and, as a teenager lost in the bliss of her world, she smiled, swaying to the sound of music.

4.2 The relationships of confusing affects

Winter was turning into Spring in Madrid, and we could go out for walks and spend more time strolling around our city's parks and plazas. We ventured into the bustling flow of people on its streets and gardens, to observe and be observed, to feel a part of the city's life, as we contemplated the trees, the budding of new leaves, as we carefully continued our work on feelings and affects together, delving into conversations of greater depth and risk. Gradually, the great emotional confusion that Yao Lu carried inside began to surface.

I knew she had a history full to the brim with maltreatment and abuse. I had been provided an outline of essential information, and I had experienced how Yao Lu lived and took-on her relationships with men as a large, confusing, and dangerous emotional entanglement. It seemed she had no understanding of the differences between a friendship, a courtship typical of boyfriends and girlfriends and most other types of relationships, or at least she had a great difficulty describing them. These differences seemed blurry to her, barely existent, and surely very far from being understood at an emotional level.

As we began talking about her experiences with the boys that appeared over the course of our work together, as well as those of her past, her profound difficulties became evident. We explored what a friend or a boyfriend was all about. She told me that a friend was a person whom one trusted more, not like a boyfriend. We explored her experiences in a couple, and with them her experiences of the *other*, the male, with whom she felt unable to speak nor share. Her relationships were not based on a foundation of trust. I had a feeling this was important to explore in our conversations. Something about these experiences would undoubtedly permeate the expectation she had of ours.

I was struck by her answer when I asked her if she had had more friends or more boyfriends in her 16-year-old life:

> More boyfriends, friends only two.

And it was her whole life she was referring to!

This part of the work was complex. We spoke about our definitions of friendship, courtships, of couples, and my own prejudices shaped each and every one of them. They were all based on my own experiences, not hers. I had been in a few romantic relationships by then, and although the degree of emotional intimacy had surely varied, I did think that a fundamental aspect in all of them was a search to share some emotional experiences, rather than being content with remaining estranged acquaintances.

To bombard Yao Lu with normative definitions and talk like a dictionary would be useless to her. She would be unable to connect with them and they would have surely made her feel more alienated than she already was. Besides, they would be definitions of my own! *We had to slowly create and question those definitions within the context of accompaniment*, as well as in her parallel psychotherapeutic treatment with her psychiatrist.

Where was intimacy in her relations with a significant other? And why was it not present in her discourse? I constructed different possibilities in my mind. And I waited. Our girl had never had a male friend, just a friend-friend, and her discourse did convey that she had had many «boyfriends» whom she was unable to count on, nor trust, experiences she felt should remain in silence. We spoke of power dynamics in relationships between couples, of barely perceptible or of egregious forms of submission; of boyfriends who bossed their girl-friends around, gave orders, commands. She remembered Marcelo, with his suffocating intrusions and her courageous capacity to break up with him, despite his unrelenting harassment.

During one of these conversations she asserted that she was no longer an «easy girl» (and in saying that she was conveying that she had been) and, intrigued by her definition, I encouraged her to de-scribe what she meant. An easy girl was one who gave in to the sexual and relational demands of the other. In contrast to the emotional intimacy worthy of a good relationship (and the idea of a *good re-lationship* cannot be but another construct of my own), an easy girl gave up sovereignty and control over herself. An easy girl was a girl removed from her very self! Where might such a perspective and *worldview* have come from?[10]

> *My task was to respect her and help her wonder about herself with enough prudence to allow for the reorganizing of her internal and relational world, without getting overwhelmed by the anxiety and insecurity that would emerge in doing so.*[11]

During those first months of my work with her, we gradually ex-plored the confusion between love and sex. She felt lost in the simi-larities and differences. She would explicitly tell me that that was her problem, that she got confused and could not tell them apart. In one of our conversations, Yao Lu asked me:

If a guy says «I love you», what does it mean?... Is that love? That's what **** told me when we had sex, but then he would leave (as she referred to a Central-American male who covered her with sugarcoated words in a syrupy voice).

I felt trapped by the binary yes/no pressure of her question. On the one hand, she was asking me about the normative definition of the words, but on the other hand, she was asking a deeper question about intimate relationships. At the same time there was a third level, she was inquiring about her experience. How was I to respond? I was about to make another mistake. Her question confounded various levels of communication that she had to untangle for herself: I was in a bind.

1   On the manifest level (content/words), she was asking for a definitive rational answer to an emotional dilemma.

2   What kind of relationship could be expected from the words «I love you»? Naïve, lost, profoundly sincere, and hopeful of being loved and to love, she was trying to figure out what love actually was. Confused by her experiences of early abuse, yet thoughtful and tentatively probing, she wanted to make sense of the behavior of that individual who left her after having sex but who spoke "words of love" inconsistent with the behavior. Yao Lu wanted to know and understand, to be able to take hold of the reins of her life.

To what was I supposed to give an answer? As an educator, as a companion, and in line with the therapeutic work of our team, the only thing I could do was to encourage her to listen to herself feel. And I was to accompany her in her search, to invite her to apprehend her own emotions. This required what Fonagy and others (Fonagy, 1991; Fonagy & Bateman, 2008; Fonagy & Target, 2006) have termed "mentalization", which was especially important when tensions were running high and relationships were so confusing.

Fonagy & Target (2006) suggest that the parent's capacity to *mentalize* the baby, involves putting themselves in their child's shoes by imagining the baby's mind and anticipating the baby's needs beyond the merely biological. This is particularly important in moments of crises, so the infant/child can feel held (imagined and understood in the mind of the other). Trust in the parental figure is fostered this way, and it also increases the child's sense of a "secure" attachment. It however requires a parent who does not have to be vigilantly monitored by the infant for the parents' own dis-regulated emotional expressions. This is predicated on (and influenced by) the parent's ability to see that the child has wishes and needs of its own. It involves a parent who, secure in themselves, who can allow for different subjectivities in the context of intersubjectivity, and for the existence of mental states in the other separate from one's own.

It turns out to be paradoxical, as Fonagy & Target (2006) further suggest, that babies or individuals with secure attachments do not feel the need to seek out attachment as frequently as a way to contain negative and overwhelming affect. In contrast, an insecurely attached child will seek out the parent, even when the parent is unavailable, or even dangerous. For example, a child whose parent unloads on him/her when coming home from a frustrating day at work, still comes to them in tears to seek comfort and security. There is no other alternative. The condition for mentalization is clearly compromised in these circumstances.

In the case of a secure relationship, as these authors hypothesize, the conditions allow for the early development of mentalization. But in order for the parent to perceive the mental states of the other, that parent must have previously experienced that kind of relationship and see oneself reflected in the other's light (Slade, 2006). That absence was very costly for Yao Lu. We can think of Yao Lu as feeling her way in the dark in search of that relationship, as was currently the case. She frequently found herself instead under the almost magnetic hypnotic spell of dissociation (Bromberg, 2003), caught in the eyes of the other where she, much like people with histories like hers, would freeze almost automatically, and submit to his/her powerful glare, as a distorted form of security.

She was trapped in the snare of the different incongruent messages (I love you and I leave you), and in asking me she ensnared me in the impossibility of the situation too. I could not give her too clear an answer. I ought not to. If I did, it would be mine only. Besides, there was no clear answer to such a tangle. More importantly, I could emphatically feel her confusion and disorientation, and that is what I had to pay attention to, instead of skipping over these difficult feelings to an "answer". Yao Lu had to build up the courage to dare to find her own emotional answer, as well as to question the relational rules that others seemed to impose on her. I had to gradually help her unveil, shed light, give legitimacy and value to her emotions- concealed, but hers nonetheless.

4.2.1 Analysis of the paradoxes and double binds

Bateson et al. (1956) coined the term *double bind* to refer to these complex messages which, in their affirmation also carry their own denial, ensnaring the receiver in the impossibility of giving a satisfactory answer. Throughout her life, Yao Lu had come across many of these messages, as was currently happening to her with men, and these were now beginning to be identified as such. Perhaps the most basic and common example of this type of communicational paradox is the following,[12] often expressed more or less subtly, by well meaning therapists:

> Be spontaneous!

The message invalidates itself, leaving the receiver trapped in an impossible situation. If one tries to be spontaneous, the person necessarily ceases to be so, and if the person does not do something different, the command goes un-obeyed. The only viable way out of this difficulty is to speak about the communication, to meta-communicate the impossibility of the message, thus stepping out of it. But this was still too much to ask of our girl. We would be able to help her interrogate these relational traps later on.

The key difficulty of a double-binding action lies in its preventing or invalidating this type of communicating about the communication. It therefore does not allow the receiver the possibility of getting out of the impossible paradox either by retracting the communication or by making the communicational dilemma explicit. That would require putting into question the speakers' authority –a difficult task for our girl.

As Watzlawick et al. (2011) made clear, pointing out the incongruous message, or the true issue at hand, is not allowed and makes matters worse. The person stuck in a double-bind is typically made to feel bad, guilty, or crazy for accurately perceiving reality. (Watzlawick et al., 2011, pp.192–193).

Would it be possible that these double binds that men put her into and that her fear of abandonment kept her trapped in, would then result in the splitting of her self and in its surrender? Very likely so.

The complexity of the double-binding messages was enormous.[13] The saccharine and cryptic words of her Central-American friend, who gifted her with psychologically abusive love, just as Marcelo's messages, helped me understand the nature of the trap I felt our girl was a prisoner to, and with which I had to work cautiously.

The following table breaks down the different levels of the contradictory and invalidating communications, each of which trapped Yao Lu, leaving her with her only default option: submission. The secondary messages were not necessarily made explicit in words (like in the case of the Central-American fellow), but were conveyed behaviorally. They were all linked to the split and emotional suppression of our girl, with its roots in the fear of being abandoned anew, and trapped by it. Did one have to suffer to such a degree in order to be loved and feel loved?

Central-American boyfriend	Marcelo
1. He would send Yao Lu two separate verbal messages: the more common and entrapping «I love you», and another that aimed at her pregnancy and helpless situation, «You need a man; you can't have your child on your own».	He said he would take charge of her son and her, that he would care for them, and occasionally he had small gifts for her.
2. Woven into these verbal messages was another behavioral one that imposed a powerful and implicit rule: «I leave whenever I'm done and whenever want to. You need a man, but I'm not that man now. You need a man, but I love you, and I'll be that man again, when I feel like it, because you need a man, but I'm leaving now because that's what I feel like doing».	He had no respect for her. It even escalated to physical abuse. The rule was that verbal care was interwoven with suffering. If she broke up with him, his menacing message was that no one would help her and she would be alone and abandoned by all since it was what she—poor thing!—in fact deserved.
3. Yao Lu's fear of abandonment made her unable to put the conflict she felt with him into words. If she did, she feared losing him. So she suppressed herself, and we had to take into account that she gained the security of having a man who described himself as necessary, albeit only when he chose to be so. With her submission and self-censorship, she was saving love.	She felt she could not talk and share with him, for her view of a couple did not include this kind of intimacy. She was an "easy girl" who did what the other wanted, "submitted" in Ghent's (1990) terms, yet always with a longing for affection. To speak of the conflict she felt with him was taboo. This way of being with men, stemmed from the abuse of her biological father, from whom she could not flee and whom she also needed in order to survive, literally. The fear of abandonment and loneliness kept her trapped. In addition, she was immobilized between the different levels of the message—care/suffering—that was then wrapped up in a suffocating blanket of fears.

Yao Lu had suffered the maltreatment and abuse of her biological father from the very beginning of her life in China. When she was barely six years old, she had mustered the courage to run away from home never to return. How might the bases of her identity have been structured in the middle of alcohol, anger, torture, hate, sex and neglect? Had love or tenderness existed there? What was love? Would affection have been withdrawn if she did not consent to the abuse? What was the meaning of sex? What kind of Dantean paradox would have loomed over a little girl whose supposed rock of stability was actually sadistic and homicidal?

When the parents' difficulties in perceiving and satisfying the child's needs are severe, as Jeremiah Abrams suggests, it paradoxically re-inforces the child's dependency. The child then develops an «as if self» that above all strives to please the parents, splitting off its incipient real self, which turns into the lost and hidden child within (Abrams, 1990, p.117). For children to be able to understand and regulate their emotions, the parents' expressions of affect must be adapted to those of the child, who then will be able to apprehend them, delineating and fleshing out their own feelings, in a relationship where both marking and mirroring are possible. This will help attach meaning to their mental states. Where marking and mirroring are absent, the symbo-lizing of experience is difficult to regulate (Fonagy & Target, 2006), mystifying and nebulous (Laing, 1965), and the resulting mental state is confusion, at best.

In the abusive relationship inflicted by her father, she would not have found the mirroring necessary to have her emotions reflected back to her. Her inner world must have been formed in an unintelligible manner, without being able to identify, let alone differentiate, her own emotions and those of the abuser who dominated and destroyed her fledgling self.

Instead, our girl adapted by splitting herself off from the abuse, so as to hold off its unbearable echoes. In order for a child to be able to create a coherent mental image of himself or herself, he or she must have first been perceived as having a mind of his or her own by his or her attachment figures (Fonagy & Target, 2006; Slade, 2006). This had not been Yao Lu's experience. Instead of rebelling—for in her early infancy she fully depended on her caretakers—she became a «good» girl (Bion, 1990): submitting to the abuse to be saved, and periodically turning all that latent aggression towards herself too. Would love thus be pain? Would suffering be necessary in the experience of love?

> That's my problem. I get confused.

Yet at the same time, Yao Lu must have perceived and felt something was not right during the earliest years of her life in China.[14] Instead of faltering and surrendering completely to her misfortune, she fled to Beijing through rice paddies with an abusive violent father in close pursuit behind her. She was a strong girl. But why did she end up reliving her misfortune with abusing men over and over again? That question resonated inside me as I accompanied her, and it was now beginning to be one she asked herself too—a good sign. Her reflective abilities were improving. We were gradually able to observe the different parts of her self and how they worked, to weave them together into a more integrated and less reactive way of being.

Trapped in those double-binding relationships, Yao Lu suppressed the part of herself pushing for change, since listening to it could be too painful and threatening. She did it with Marcelo, when faced with his threats of abandonment; she did it with the Central American male who wooed her with sickly-sweet words - «I love you, my love» – but then abandoned her as if she were an object of no value. She would do so with other men, before this malignant and vicious circle of hers would begin to crumble. She was trapped amongst chaotic emotions and confusing messages that kept her in a constant whirlwind with men, each one of whom made her feel victimized once again, and she was incapable of separating herself from them due to the terrifying fear of loneliness.

Right about this time, Yao Lu's pregnancy entered into its second trimester.

Notes

1 Adopted children can carry a primary injury inflicted by the abandonment by their biological parents who could not, did not know how to, or simply did not want to take care of them. This narcissistic injury frequently resonates in all subsequent losses.

2 Levin (1993) describes narcissistic injuries as pains that loom over us when our identity, self-image, self-esteem, or ego-ideal are under threat; pains that resonate in the depths of our being, unleashing feelings of shame, humiliation, and rage.

3 For further understanding and case examples of these dynamics within family systems, the reader is invited to look into Harriet Lerner's (1989) book «The Dance With Anger»—Chapter 8—from which the ideas here were adapted to understand and improve interventions between educators and children in care. Lerner explains how it is helpful to get detailed histories of the parents' families of origin, since they may be affecting the reactions and triangular formations surfacing in each particular stage of the family's life cycle, which may be triggered by parental experiences from their own past.

4 Berliner, B. B. (1958) p.46. «The role of object relations in moral masochism.» *Psychoanalytic Quarterly*, 27, 38–56.

5 For more information on the differences between submission and surrender we invite the reader to the seminal article by Ghent (1990), «Masochism, submission, surrender...», where masochism is described as a perversion of surrender. Surrender for Ghent does not involve defeat in the sense of capitulation to the other, but has to do with an expansion of the self, in which, as one's own defenses diminish and loosen-up, one feels more whole, enriched and liberated through the meeting of subjectivities. It is very different from submission, which involves a voluntary resignation of wishes and subjectivity to the benefit of another. Surrender, therefore, is not voluntary, cannot be controlled, but instead involves a «letting go», a discovery in-and-with the other, and thus has a quality of expansiveness and growth in the encounter.

6 D.W. Winnicott (1971) likens psychotherapy as two people who are at play together. When that does not happen, the therapists' goal [in this case the therapeutic companion] is to help the patient get there. (p.38).

7 Mitchell made a constructive critique of what he described as "pragmatic dissociations" in classical psychoanalysis, which helped analysts manage the intensity of the clinical encounter, placing them out of an intersubjective relationship that could not only make use of them, but that was also a part of them. For him, the therapeutic relationship was much more similar to other human relationships than what Freud would have liked, and he suggested that it was precisely in the inter-subjectivity and the participant patient-therapist relationship where change would take place (p.125). In this sense he positioned himself within the relationship, influencing and being influenced by it, comparable to the systems therapists from the second-order cybernetics and constructivist and social constructionist perspectives.

8 S. Mitchell (2010), referring to H. Loewald, described the inextricable link between the intersubjective context and the development of an individual mind and subjectivity (p.57). In other words, there is no «me» without a «you», and no individual without someone who constructs it in the relationship. Mitchell was not denying the development of the individual mind, but he was suggesting that those spaces arise from the intersubjective matrix, and are experienced as

subjective experiences of one's own, within an interpersonal field where the qualities and motivations of an individual subjectivity gradually emerge. From this vantage point, the mind cannot be other than something that arises, forged in an internalized interpersonal field. Personal properties and experiences are generated, regulated, and transformed by the same interpersonal matrix they are part of, in dynamics of internal and external interactional-regulation. That is, the individual cannot exist without its world and the relationships that create it. And I was now in Yao Lu's world myself, just as much as she had become a part of mine. At times these emotions emerging in the relationship, and the emotional containment of Yao Lu was complex and it affected me more than I liked to admit. It was important for me to take care of myself as well, and that was what my supervision was for, to a large extent.

9 Bucay, J. (2013): *Let me tell you a story: Tales along the road to happiness*, New York, Europa Editions. [Original in Spanish (2002): *Déjame que te cuente: Los cuentos que me enseñaron a vivir*, Barcelona, RBA Libros].

10 Making use of Ghent's (1990) terms, an easy girl would be a submissive one, and Yao Lu's submission seemed to have the hints of a longing, of a quest for her self, in which her masochism was a means "to save love through suffering" (Berliner, 1958, p.46 in Caflisch, 2012; or in *Psychoanalytic Quarterly*, 27, 38–56). In the complementarity of identity formation in a submissive relation, there also seemed to be the elements of an encounter, of a re-encounter with the parts of her *self* that had been diluted in the relationship with the other: what Bromberg (1996) addressed as dissociated self-states. The tsunami of affective hyperarousal and its complicated regulation (Bromberg, 2008) made these states inaccessible through language. Bromberg (2003, 2008) pointed out the importance of reducing the patients' vulnerability to affective hyperarousal through therapeutic 'safe surprises', where risk, though it does not cease to exist, is moderated by a relationship that includes both subjectivities, that does not privilege one at the expense of the other. Similarly, Fonagy (1991), Fonagy & Target (2006), and Fonagy & Bateman, (2008) described the serious difficulties patients diagnosed with borderline personality disorder have self-regulating and reflecting on their and others' mental states, thoughts, intentions, and feelings. This difficulty seems to have its roots in their early attachments, and these authors advocate for an approach attuned to the vicissitudes of attachment, especially when the challenges of emotional hyperarousal arise. Yao Lu, in states of hyperarousal, fear, and anxiety would seek out a sexual relationship with a man to whom she could be and remain submitted as a way to regulate her hyperarousal. In this submission she found security, or at least its simulation.

11 Yao Lu had also spent the first long years of her life in China, where rigid constructs of gender and cultural identity had already been partially formed in her young life. In her therapeutic work with first-generation Chinese immigrants born in the United States, B. Eisold (2012) found many struggled to assert their own needs, or even identify them, when those challenged familial expectations (p.239). In reference to A. Roland (1996), an author she speaks about in her

article, she suggests that Asian families develop a *we-self*, in contrast to the individuality of the western *I-self*. A. Roland describes the we-self as a less assertive one, more interwoven in interdependencies and needs of the other. One's own needs are not made explicit, and are found in longings for empathic connection. There is an assumption that they are seen in relation to another without having to verbalize their needs, in a web ruled by hierarchies of gender and cultural obedience. Might this have something to do with Yao Lu's dynamics with the men in her life, who were older and authoritarian?

12 The example, although likely a common one echoing in classrooms and academic contexts attempting to describe the double-bind, was taken from the Pragmatics of Human Communication (p.220).

13 The original article by Bateson et al. (1956) titled: «Toward a theory of Schizophrenia», described a communicational dynamic common to families with a schizophrenic member. Although in this day and age, the weight of genetic factors in the pathogenesis of the illness is generally accepted, double-binding communicational relations continue to shed light on many tense intra-family and interpersonal dynamics. These authors flesh out the double bind into six fundamental parts: 1) the existence of an intense relationship between two or more people; 2) the recurrence of the communications; 3) punishment for both complying and not complying. The interpersonal message, incongruent in its different communicational levels—be it punishment in the form of abandonment, emotional withdrawal, or the expression of anger—would usually be verbal in content; 4) another of the incongruences is conveyed non-verbally—whether through the cadence in a voice, one's physical posture in relation to another, etc., which would be disconfirming of the content of the verbal message—or with a verbal message that was incongruent in content such as «Be spontaneous», or «I love you but I make you feel bad/I am abusing/I make you feel pain»; 5) the imposition of a third incongruent imperative, which would not allow for the person to exit the trap by making explicit—metacommunicating—that responding to all the levels of the message was an impossibility. This imperative could be the result of a threat of rejection or of an outright prohibition, which, in Yao Lu's case, would be a threat to her very survival given her complete dependence on her primary figures in infancy; and, later, this dynamic was repeated in the promised love of her maltreating boyfriends; and 6) once this habitual dynamic is entrenched the whole sequence is no longer necessary in order to see the world in double binds. The emergence of any part of the sequence is sufficient to activate in full. (adaptation from the original article, pp. 6 & 7).

14 To get a novelized idea of female experience, possibly similar to Yao Lu's in her early years in China, the reader is invited to read Xinran's *Message from an unknown Chinese mother* (2010). The novel captures the experiences of abandonment and infanticide of unwanted Chinese girls, and the emotional submission of women to sociocultural pressure that includes the devalued gender construct of women.

Chapter 5

Second trimester's wait: Where do we come from?

5.1 The therapeutic accompaniment system as a fluctuating space

My accompaniment was nestled at the juncture of different personal histories and cultures that echoed within the space of our relationship. We encountered each other at the intersection of two particular worldviews, which set the parameters for us to influence each other. Yao Lu brought a set of unconscious and lived experiences (constructs) to our relationship; her relations with men, her experiences in China and Spain, and her expectations with other male caretakers in her life. I added my own constructs and lived experience from childhood and adolescence into the equation, and even without being directive—at times without even being aware of it—I induced Yao Lu into slight modifications of her world, in a transactional dyad of reciprocating experience, a shared one, though we both had different ways of experiencing it (Figure 5.1). This did not involve mutuality in the sense of reciprocal causality, but a contribution of us both—we were both co-creating a relationship, which was emerging between us—although, due to the nature of my work, I was contributing to a different degree (Beebe & Lachman, 1998). This was an asymmetric complementarity then; while the relationship influenced me equally, it required of me a greater degree of self-awareness and self-regulation in processing both of our emotions.[1] It was necessary to be aware of the constructs and experiences that shaped our different ways of experiencing the world. Though our realities were different, they could be compatible, and the therapeutic system we created could work (Elkaïm, 1997, p. 69).

DOI: 10.4324/9781003261490-5

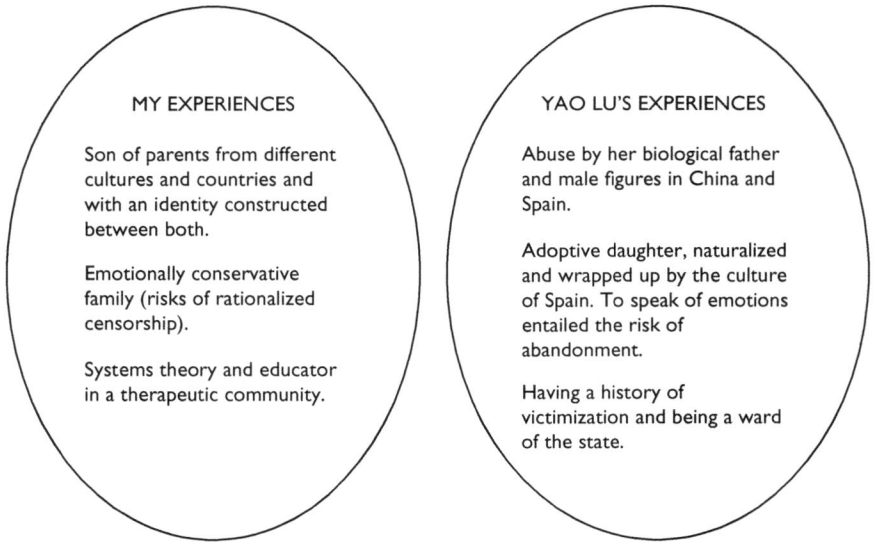

MY EXPERIENCES

Son of parents from different
cultures and countries and
with an identity constructed
between both.

Emotionally conservative
family (risks of rationalized
censorship).

Systems theory and educator
in a therapeutic community.

YAO LU'S EXPERIENCES

Abuse by her biological father
and male figures in China and
Spain.

Adoptive daughter, naturalized
and wrapped up by the culture
of Spain. To speak of emotions
entailed the risk of
abandonment.

Having a history of
victimization and being a ward
of the state.

Figure 5.1 Two different worldviews.

Obviously, Yao Lu did not keep all of this in mind. That responsibility
was mine.

Our relationship provided the space for these foundational experiences to emerge, and hopefully to change, though not before they
would be repeated, to some extent. For instance, if I unconsciously
sought her smiles as a balm for the injuries to my own pride, or
pressured her to provide me with recognition for my job and work as
a therapeutic companion, I would run the risk of feeding into and
reinforcing her worldview. In it, the male, an emotionally distant
authoritarian, always demanded that others answer to his own wishes
and needs.

If I were blinded and dominated by my own narcissistic needs I
would also be incapable of perceiving the hidden and real Yao Lu,
unknown even to herself, as she would adapt to fit my own hidden
longings, in a self-suppressing attempt to please me (Green, 1980;
Miller, 1981), thus repeating her constricted and insecure relations
with men. This would push her to remain in the darkness of her split-
off world, from where it was so necessary she emerge. I had to at least
try to be aware of this; I had to be conscious of my abilities and

shortcomings, so that I would not burden her as much with them. This would allow her to grow (incrementally) in the relationship, instead of repeating yet again a relationship in which she was forced to go into hiding, and of trivializing her insoluble pain in the process (represented in Figure 5.2 by the thick arrow followed by the arrow of dashes).

In my therapeutic role, I took on the delicate task of challenging and deconstructing her worldview, while carefully avoiding the traps that would reinforce that worldview. A new dance that veered away from the usual expectations of her life, would allow for the construction of a new relational reality (represented by the thick arrow and the dotted arrow in Figure 5.2).

But at the same time, Yao Lu demanded of me firmness and clear boundaries, to deal not just with her temperamental outbursts but also with her submissive proposals, from which I had to disentangle myself without being hurtful, while also managing to validate her experience so as to construct a genuine relationship. If unsuccessful, I would lead her (and me) once again into a paradoxical knot. My

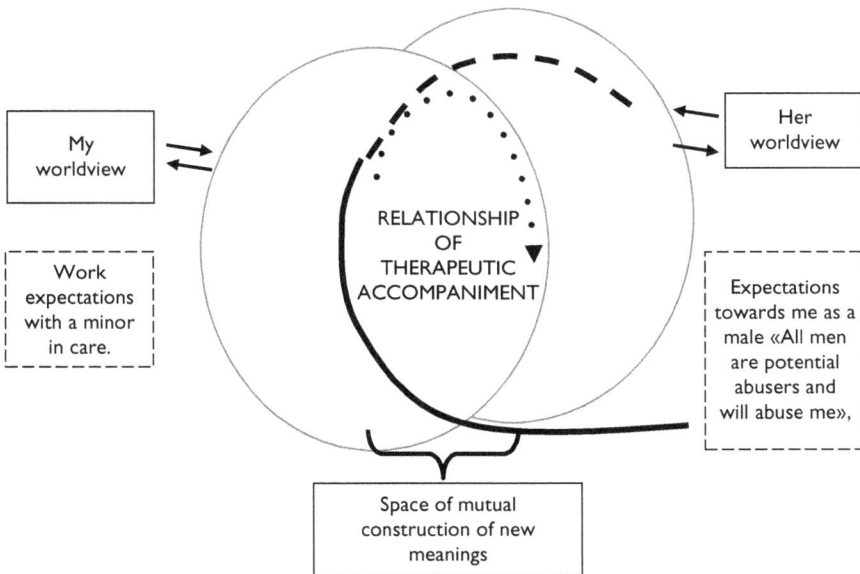

Figure 5.2 Constellation of two worldviews in a system of therapeutic accompaniment.

influence over her was matched by the risk of alienating her and of her fleeing into her inner world. In my desire to help her there lay the risk of coercing her, and thus impeding her change, which would bring her right back to her negative construct of men. This made the serene and respectful therapeutic alliance crucial for a new and different relational space to emerge, one absent of submission.[2]

In addition, reflecting on my own images of Yao Lu was necessary, given that the ideas I may have had of her were just as important as the ones she may have had of me; they both determined the nature of our relationship. I saw *Yao Lu as a girl capable of taking ownership of her life responsibly, a strong girl.* I held this vision, even in the midst of constant instability of her emotional storms.

5.2 Work outside the therapeutic setting

5.2.1 The soothing connection and reassuring places

Both Yao Lu and the space we were gradually constructing asked for a serene, welcoming, and relaxed maternal posture from me. Thus I absorbed her anxieties, providing serenity and security in return, to support and help her face the storm of her dreaded feelings.

As time and the seasons passed by, the seeds of this work began to take root and we were able to explore the depths of her memories and experiences. Protected by our frame, our conversations started to bloom during our walks in the park amongst the new leaves and flowers. Yao Lu's belly was also growing, as was the curiosity of those who looked at us in the street. I dared not touch her belly to avoid any confusion, even if she had invited me to do so. Perhaps it was to avoid the anxiety of feeling the beating of a life «more alive» inside her, which was also under my care. In this «technical rationalization», I was excluding one of the fundamental ways to relate with others—touch. It was not until the possibility of my latent fears were brought up in my supervision, that I was able to disentangle myself from my own intellectualized defenses—to then relate in a more natural way. Nevertheless, I never did touch her belly, nor was it ever recommended.

We must have been quite a sight. I remember very vividly one day when, after we walked up the steps to the subway platform, I briefly stopped to tie my shoelaces as Yao Lu went on walking to sit on an empty bench she spotted at the far end. Overriding the city rule to look past your neighbor, nearly every one of the seventy or so people waiting for the train followed Yao Lu with their gaze. It was as if a powerful magnet were compelling them to turn their necks; one after the other, like a row of dominos, their stares centered on our very adolescent, and very pregnant, Chinese girl. They were transfixed by awe, for a few seconds, before they pulled themselves back together to look out into the emptiness before them again, as if awoken from a dream.

But it was neither a dream nor a mirage, it was something very real. I vividly recall the whispered words of one lady to another, as a musical undertone: «Take a look at that one with the bun in the oven!». I ignored them and walked on to sit at her side. What might have been going on in the minds of those motley travelers on that platform?—Fears, prejudice, rejections, tenderness?

Yao Lu, the teenager that she was, walked down the streets of stigma. She was pregnant and she was Chinese. At a time when the Asian population was incorporating itself into the cultural and ethnic richness of our country, public eyes scrutinized her closely (Goffman, 1986). We had to maneuver in and around the public stigma. Goffman reflects on the intricacies and impediments of living under the stigmatizing scrutiny of others. I certainly had the urge to confront the stares and prejudices, and expose their ignorance, of a small yet great Other—our pregnant girl. What did they know about the tormented life of the one they freely passed judgment on? It was an injustice!

It was neither the first nor the last time I would have to deal with public preconceptions of her and of me. When Yao Lu got herself into some major mess, or she was nowhere to be found and I feared danger, I would be torn between what to share and what not to share when I looked for her. I asked about her and was met with suspicious stares. People had their doubts about me, and about her. I would introduce myself as an educator searching for her, reluctantly revealing her situation as a pregnant minor under the care of the state. I was repeatedly forced to decide what to say, and to whom.

Little by little, we began creating a web of sorts, of reliable contacts, of good Samaritans, to whom I responded in subtle evasions when faced with having to reveal her history or the reasons for my accompanying her. But some people did understand, and they would help protect her.

Yao Lu was beginning to be aware of the curiosity she sparked around her, it could be read in the eyes of passers-by scanning her until they reached her incipient belly. Back then she identified with Juno,[3] as we tried to learn from her character.

> That woman checked me out because I'm pregnant. [...] My mother always says «Cover up! Cover up!», and I tell her «C'mon Mom no, it doesn't matter. Besides you are going to be able to tell anyway»...

Instead of feeling like she had to hide herself, she should stand tall and keep walking towards a life free from the torments of the past. And that was how she walked before the crowd on the platform, courageously. This was how we worked, conversing out in the open, some days on the terraced area of a tranquil cafeteria, others in a park surrounded by the chirping of birds, and it felt like the world's music was revolving around us.

She was feeling harbored in the shelter of our relationship. With the strength it gave her, she dipped into difficult memories. We spoke then of her experiences in our Therapeutic Community and her journey getting there, of the situation of other children she had gotten to know, of their particular itineraries, and indirectly of her own.

> The thing is some have had problems in their childhood and of course ... they're not doing well.
> So ... Having or not having a happy childhood, with fond memories, can have something to do with the way people act?
> Hmmm ... yea.
> And have you had a happy childhood, with happy memories? [And a silence emerged, which I allowed, long and caring, respectful and serene, for I understood that even without an answer, the memories were arising ... and a short while later she moved her head in a slow and silent «No»].
> I've been an abused child. My biological father raped me, and one in Spain did too.

She began narrating her story. Paradoxically, while Yao Lu allowed herself to share her *traumatic memories*, the scenery outside was of a radiant Spring day.

She told me how in China she had spent most of her time locked up in a room, captive to a drunken father, and how she had attempted an escape through a broken window. When she managed to get out, she usually stumbled upon him and received a thrashing. She was an only child, and at that time the news broadcasts in our country echoed with girls tied to the chairs of orphanages. It was very likely that this man, who might have wished for a male child from his wife in order to be the proud patron of a respectable family in the eyes of his rural culture, poured his rage onto the most innocent member as he saw his future crumble with the birth of little Yao Lu. Had he tried to kill her? Probably, and perhaps his deadly wish had been frustrated by a mother who refused to have her daughter's life come to a tragic end. Maybe it was then that a triad of violence, alcohol, and ever-present death took hold. As objectified subjects of patriarchal traditions made to satisfy the narcissistic needs of men, women were not worth much at all, and if they were unable to give birth to a male child, worth even less.

She recalled how, on one occasion, her father grabbed her by the head and plunged her repeatedly in a pail of dirty water to drown her, and she mimicked the scene to show me. One could understand where her present anxiety about swimming underwater in the pool came from, or why she didn't like the deep end. It made her feel out of breath. She described her experience by using the universal gesture of gripping her neck with both hands. Further along, she would mention, in another soul-wrenching story, how her father would hang her up from her legs to beat her, or would force her to eat her own feces. Just hearing it made one's gut churn. But she had actually lived this nightmare.

Our conversation then drifted to happier times of a recent vacation by the sea, as if her surging memories needed a less emotionally threatening association to settle them. I was not to press her, but to just be there and listen to whatever it was she wanted to or was able to speak about. In this to and fro, between trauma and safety, like the waves on a beach, we built a safe harbor.

Yao Lu was beginning to feel sheltered, and in that protected world, hope bloomed anew. Just before we got up from the bench, she said:

> I think this year is going to be a very good one and then it'll be like that forever... I'm just sure now.

And we had just navigated through the treacherous seas of her terrifying experiences!

Yao Lu was feeling a gentle ray of hope. She wanted to relive her childhood with us, but this time, as she said herself, a «happy childhood». The times were turbulent, yet hopeful, calm yet stormy, sunny amidst April rains. But in the middle of new flowerbeds, weeds still reappear.

Notes

1   Fogel (1992) came to describe this relational system as one of co-regulation, where behavior taking place in the individual is having an impact, and thus influencing and being influenced by the behavior of the other at the same time (referred to in the article «Co-constructing inner and relational processes-self and mutual regulation in infant research and adult treatment» Beebe & Lachman, 1998. Fogel's seminal article provides a deeper description of the concept and his thinking: Fogel, A. 1992. «Movement and communication in human infancy: the social dynamics of development» *Human Movement Science*, 11, 387–423). Similarly, Fonagy & Target (2006) define affective regulation—in our case a dyadic co-regulation—as the capacity of modulating emotional or affective states. From their perspective, this regulation is a necessary prelude to the development of the capacity to mentalize—so necessary and complex in the case of Yao Lu—and then to think of others in terms of their mental states, and to reflect about one's self in terms of mood, affect, and emotion. Mentalization will not only serve as a way of regulating affect, but also of regulating the *self* per se.
2   For an excellent study of the gender-based difficulties one must bear in mind when involved in psychotherapeutic activity, and of ways for intervening, please see the article: «Beyond different worlds: A "post-gender" approach to relational development» (C. Knudson-Martin and A.R. Mahoney (1999).
3   Yao Lu was now remembering the lead character in the film *Juno* (directed by Jason Reitman and written by Diablo Cody in 2007) which we had seen months before, and she identified with her, since she was living similar experiences that were gradually weaving themselves into her daily life, reducing the feeling of alienation in a world that could thus begin to have meaning for her. Her belly went on growing as did people's curiosity.

Chapter 6

Third trimester's wait:
Problems in communication

6.1 Traps and paradoxes of abuse: The communicative significance of play

6.1.1 Recollections of Peter Pan and strategies towards an implicit dialogue

For several days, Yao Lu made herself unavailable, a sort of spring-like instability. Soon, I found myself probing the Internet yet again until I stumbled upon one of her recent messages searching for new friends. This time, it was less revealing. Nonetheless, sending out messages and telephone numbers into the open world of the Web still constituted a big risk.

One morning, when I was arriving at the train station near the maternity home, I saw her sitting on the opposite platform, absorbed in her thoughts. Once again, I had the feeling that, though she had been avoiding me, Yao Lu was waiting for me there.

I went over to her and let her know of my concern without dumping my anxieties on her, but showing her my affection and interest in her wellbeing. She had disappeared for a few days. I brought up what I had been thinking, accompanied by humor in my tone— «Might she be hiding? Nooo, it couldn't be»—and when her hard expression cracked with a chuckle, I invited her to a hot chocolate since it was a cold day.[1] I then became more directive in my tone, feeling that her resistances gave way to laughter.

As we warmed up with our cups of hot chocolate, we ventured into an almost artistic bobbin-laced dialogue, threaded with the under-currents of emotions we attempted to elude. We were on a quest to

DOI: 10.4324/9781003261490-6

reconnect, but it was a reconnection laden with feelings of turmoil and sadness that were hidden behind her distant, evasive, and passive gaze. Like the Impressionist painter whose work only gains clarity as he moves along, we began to talk. Yao Lu would be able to come back to the mothering relationship if she so wished, like the children in *Neverland* in the tale of Peter Pan (Barrie, 1911), whose mother always left the windows of their home open, welcoming and expecting their possible return.

I asked how she had been, but it did not take us far; her lips pursed and quivered as if she were keeping control of the turbulent emotional struggle within. Dark secrets pushing towards daylight, as there were fears of being judged. These fears invited her to hide, in the paradoxically comforting darkness of pain and solitude, where there was less risk of being reprimanded anew. I kept this firmly in mind.

I gradually created a game, to which she unknowingly invited me, where I stuck to rules I had to learn and that would "allow" her to communicate. I took on my role as a naïve searcher—and in a way, that was what I was—who unsuccessfully walked around parks, streets, plazas, and Internet cafes; somewhat dazed and confused by my own bewilderment. I said: «I'm such a terrible searcher!», she chuckled and, at the same time, gifted me with small pearls of information—«I wasn't around here. I was down-town!»—which helped me comprehend my amusing incompetence better, because Yao Lu had not even been in the neighborhood in which I had been looking for her.

We constructed the rules of a non-invasive game that allowed her to speak of what she would not otherwise be able to, as we both paused in that tranquil cafeteria. I asked her if she had gone alone or with someone, and she laughed as an answer, abandoning herself to the fun of watching me guess. She would not have wandered too far on her own! So I then went on to ask about the mysterious companion, and how she had found him—«Like this?»—as I looked under the napkin dispenser; and once again she burst into loud delighted laugher.

I was leaving the world of adults to speak to her within that of children, in search of a connection that would allow her/us to communicate. As an adult immersed in the universe of the little ones, I had to be open to new and imaginative forms of communication. This opened the gates to a different world in which her fears could be expressed more easily.

In games such as these, one reconnects with the *inner child* frequently forgotten under the burden of our adult responsibilities. It is a kind of conscious journey to unconscious recollections; to the world of fantasies, dreams and imaginations lost, to recover them and to speak through them. E. Berne (1975) wrote about this when he outlined transactional analysis. As a therapeutic companion, it was necessary to reconnect to the world of children[2] lost as they may be in the castle of their fears, and invite them to play in the light of a new dawn. This required that I remain playfully connected to myself too. Playing is an essential form of communication, and in the play we were speaking without really doing so, of what would otherwise be inaccessible.

Nevertheless, it occurred to me to ask about the name of the companion, and a blanket of fog settled over us as if in a fairytale, silence ruling yet again in protective withdrawal. That question was based on my adult rules, bound to a world of logic and reason, not to that of emotion, to which the world of children is much closer. My hastiness broke the rules. I backpedaled and brought her back to her pace and the rules of our game. «Man, that was a terrible question! I didn't like it. Let's see, I'll give it another shot … Hmm… Was it a boy? … because today seems more like a day for single word answers, right?». And Yao Lu answered in a verbal and clear «yes». It was a boy.

Through a childish game, we unveiled what was otherwise not so frivolous. «Wow, wow, wow, this is awesome. This is like that game of "Guess who?". Remember that game that was like "He has blue eyes and a beard? Hmmm … It's Lucas!"», I said lifting up a sugar packet and pretending as if the game were on the table.

We started sketching a story through an imaginary game of riddles placed on the table before us, as she guided me with her answers for the novice player that I was. After a while, I guessed the identity hidden behind fearful secrets. Marcelo, the man from the Internet whose promises of protection were wrapped in pain, was back.

6.1.2 Lost emotions, externalizing and alternative narratives

Yao Lu catapulted herself back into her protective withdrawal when I guessed the secret identity. With the care of a surgeon, picking my way between a frivolous game and all too serious questions, I then started to explore how Marcelo had managed to see her again. Her mouth was trembling, her lips quivering as she got to the brink of tears—but cry she did not.

She regained control of her feelings and I calmed her down with soothing words. I hoped she would regain her ability to talk to me. She broke her silence, and amidst the bustling crowd, she started to tell me how Marcelo and his saccharine-sweet words had persuaded her to meet him again.

Yao Lu, striving for self-protection, had passed herself off as a friend of hers when she spoke to him over the phone. Her strategy involved introducing an alter-ego "her friend", who could say what she could not. Disguised as she was, she called him out on having behaved badly, and told him that Yao Lu did not want to see him ever again. She also let him know that she was really angry. But he, cunning and sly, had answered that he was heartbroken. He played her well, yet it seemed that the usually split-off emotional part of her—suppressed in the abusive relationships with men—was trying to stand, protectively, but the adolescent she was felt unable to.

So we spoke about this «friend with the good advice» who had protected and accompanied her when meeting Marcelo previously. Through this fictional companion, the exploration of her experience was more bearable. I turned into an ally of that protective and fighting part of herself that was sometimes hidden but could still be found.

We sat down once again as fellow explorers to navigate her internal world. She felt lonely, or at least my intuition told me that, and maybe there was something we could do about it.

Lonely, but a little accompanied. [She was answering to what my intuition sensed was evident and nodding in agreement with her slightly trembling fingers].

Aha, so is Loneliness to blame here? Is it as if Loneliness had come along yesterday and had said, «shut up Yao Lu's friend», or «Yao Lu, go meet Marcelo»?

Yea, somewhat. [Thus Loneliness turned into something more external, more tangible, and workable in the playfulness of language since in Spanish Loneliness (*Soledad*) is also a woman's name].

That darned Soledad! I really don't like her! [And Yao Lu began to smile, nodding in assent while she looked at me, looked at the ground, then up, and responded again in a gestural «Yes»].

Well, I think we have quite a few tools to give Soledad the boot. Boy did that sound classy! To give her the boot! Let me rephrase that, you have many ways to give Soledad's a big ol' kick in the ass! [I performed the mimicry sending off a kick into the air, to where our enemy "Loneliness" would have been, personified by now as Soledad in the imagination we shared, and Yao Lu burst into laughter]. Besides, for starters you have our psychiatrist, all the members of our team, and me. But on top of that, would you like to have friends your age?

Yes. [This was another crucial aspect of her anxiety and worry, chronically beset by the lonesome effects of Soledad].

Well, come on then. And I'll help you kick Soledad around a little, so you can fight her. We'll help you, and someday you'll find people your age. [And Yao Lu, smiling more, joined in the pummeling of the air in the fight against our fictional enemy who was so present and real in her world].

Yao Lu was caught in a turbulence of emotions, fueled by that darned Soledad that affected me as well. After all, I was also working alone; alone on the street and in the day-to-day work with Yao Lu. In referring to «the Loneliness» (i.e. Soledad),[3] we were externalizing it (White & Epston, 1990) so we could see with a new perspective. It brought us both together. Thus we constructed a protective alliance, which took care of Yao Lu and allowed us both to intensify our relationship through our shared experience. It allowed us to speak about profound feelings without being flooded by them. Instead of plunging into the torments of the emotion, we turned it into an external object with a name. It was a sort of tactical-narrative movement in the battle against her persistent enemy. We joined in a coalition against this Soledad, a companion to both of us. We identified Soledad's lurking presence in her relationships with men, a feeling she seldom spoke about. She was in a new relationship now, at least to some extent; watched over by me, a male and an educator—a different type of man—one who thought her feelings were important.

Soledad was a significant problem, and to the extent that "her" effects disappeared, so did she, for Soledad—a.k.a. loneliness—could not survive without them. One could say that the problem relied on its effects to survive (White & Epston, 1990, p.63). We had to disentangle Yao Lu's relationship with Soledad, we had to undermine the problem, by offering alternatives she might find in her relationship with me. In understanding her relationship with Soledad, we might also minimize its effects on her; and the process itself would help Yao Lu not feel so lonesome.

We worked to connect with the hopes of a new and different world, in the emerging narrative of her own. It gave her the green light to fight and allowed for the projection of a better world.

In his seminars and writing, Viktor Frankl (1962, 1968), as many others, invited people to reflect on the human being's need to search for purpose and meaning in life, and to have others believe in them, in order to live up to their true potential. While taking Yao Lu back to the recurrent story of her life was necessary, being stuck in it darkened her path; the new narratives threw up a blanket of stars that lit up her darkness with hopes. Believing in her was necessary, so she could believe, fight, and build herself. I did believe in her, as did our entire team. It was through the stories and narratives, and through the varied forms of playfulness, which redefined hopes, that profound and hidden strengths, intrinsic to her existence and life, began to assert themselves.

6.1.3 The protection and sacrifice of speechlessness and the pain of listening to oneself feel

To move beyond her history of deeply problematic relationships with men and with Soledad was a difficult, almost impossible, task. She let me know this by disappearing. This was also a time of conflict with her mother. We sensed that, in spite of everything, Marcelo continued to have a strong hold on her, using syrupy sweetness to exploit her with his ally Soledad and her army of abandonment fears.

One day Yao Lu showed up with conspicuous «hickies» on her neck. They were almost bruises. When I looked at her she responded, «I don't know». Her evasiveness, resistance, and fears were reactivated. She said nothing. Once again, we resumed our safe game of «Guess Who?», and soon enough we could recognize the tracks the same evildoer had left behind. Marcelo moved in the shadows of silence.

I knew this psychopathic individual had our girl trapped. One day, my gut churned with acid after our girl appeared with marks on her neck again. She told me with open angst that he had made them; that she had told him not to, but that he had answered that it was *so her educators would see*. Her educators! That is... Me! My blood boiled.

I had to stay as calm as possible but be tough at the same time, direct and sharp, but also cunning and sly with respect to this un-desirable abuser. I tried to get Yao Lu to understand the potential catastrophe and to push him aside. My paternalism was activated. Our girl was in danger.

This individual, who on the one hand gave her small gifts regularly, had on the other hand taken over her phone's memory card, he controlled our adolescent through insistent nocturnal calls bolstered by the threat of telling her mother how they met.

Moreover, he had charmed her mother with beguiling words and promises of protection for the girl, seemingly more from a manip-ulative desire to please the mother and obtain some material benefit, than from an affectionate attitude. Since the mother-daughter re-lationship was so conflicted, Marcelo was able to «sneak into» the gap between them and feel right at home.

I searched for information on this guy online, through the telephone number Yao Lu had given me. It was alarming. Through that number, I came upon email addresses, other cellphones, his curriculum vitae, his picture, and his real name and ID; and with an endless list of adver-tisements where he «rented» his physical attributes for a price (I will spare the reader these more crude descriptions) as well as numerous pages of loving contacts where he portrayed himself in poetry as a caring, romantic and sweet person. It was awful! But, from whose perspective? Would Yao Lu be able to see it?

He did not mix his telephone numbers: one for each different persona, but that was not the case with his email addresses; those did intermingle with the numbers. At the time I felt like, and was, a detective, in addition to an educator.

Yao Lu protected herself in a steady and impenetrable «I don't know» when we questioned her. Speaking was still too painful. At this point in our work, I could allow myself to be more incisive. After five months of calming, of containing, and of reconnecting our girl through our relationship of accompaniment, she allowed me that. Progressively, my posture had begun to shift towards a more conventionally paternal figure, leaning on my prior maternal position. Yao Lu now needed firmness and security, a stable ground to lean on. She was reshaping herself in relation to others through the growing trust in our relationship. I persisted in my inquiry, in incisive but tactful ways that conveyed my care, and our girl collapsed into tears.

> My problems are the relationships with boys.

As so she did, the lifting of the burden she felt allowed for the previously childish, flirtatious, distant, and protective shield to make way for a sad, hurt little girl to emerge through the tears. Yao Lu told me that every time she attempted to tell him she would have nothing to do with him, Marcelo convinced her to go out and to continue the relationship.

The protective mutism had spared our adolescent from the fullness of her emotions, but it was false protection gained at too high a price. She buried both fears and hopes, and so harmed herself as much as she protected herself. She said she did not even feel attracted to him. I pointed to her resentment of him, reminding her how one day, harsh and impassive, he had told her not to wear a miniskirt because she was provoking people and he didn't want to see her like that. Yet the next day he partially undressed her publicly in the street, thus underlining the contradictory message that sets up the parameters of an abusive relationship.[4]

I suggested she would have to think about whether she was willing to sacrifice herself like that, relinquishing her freedom and the control of her life to Marcelo. Her eyes dampened yet again, her defensive façade crumbling. I guided her back to a definition of herself as a strong, good, and resilient fighter. She did not deserve a guy like that, because he was a «douchebag»—and thus I took her back to words, and feelings, of the *therapeutic triangulation* of our past game—and pointed out that we all were by her side and would be there to help her out of the gauntlet. I felt it necessary to build her up, in order for her to have the confidence to handle the physical and psychic pain of her relationship with Marcelo, while at the same time being there in case she fell. In order to free herself from the prison of dissociated emotions, Yao Lu needed to listen to her feelings without opening up a new wound; so she could feel held and not revictimized by my concerned inquiries and suggestions.

I attentively read her non-verbal messages, easing up when I saw she connected to the feelings trapped inside. Here I would help her regain her strength and courage to face the pain and to keep her intolerable anxieties at bay. It was obvious she was trapped in a difficult and tormenting situation, from which she found it hard to escape. I suggested that if she wanted, and only if she wanted, I could go with her the next time she met Marcelo, but only as support; it was she who would have to do the talking. She chose to go on her own then. Truth be told, I thought it was really the only way. If she was not ready, my going with her would only turn me into a degraded puppet before this individual. Yao Lu could run even greater risks then, faced with his fury on later occasions when I would no longer be present. I certainly had the desire to meet him, even more after unmasking him on the Internet. A meeting like the one I was envisioning, was not ideal... nor the most therapeutic!

By my next visit, Yao Lu had faced the uncertainty of her fears, and wound up in the hospital about to lose her baby.

Yao Lu felt lost, having no awareness or knowledge of what a caring and affectionate relationship with a man might be like. As she would eventually tell me, she had asked a friend to tell Marcelo to «go to hell», but after insistent text messages, he managed to see her the next day, waiting for her at the entrance of the maternity home. Yao Lu gave him back his things, but he insisted on staying; he touched her, caressed her, and tricked her until he got her to have sexual intercourse, out in the open, over a handrail on the stairs that were now painted with the drops of her blood, which she showed me while narrating her failed attempt to take a stand.

When she had started to bleed, Marcelo with the coldness of a psychopath, told her to get dressed and leave. She did so, leaving a trail of red stains on the ground behind her. He would call her later that night to ask if it was serious—stark, chilling, and indifferent.

But how could it be that our young 16-year-old could remain unmoved while showing and telling me a tale of horror, framed by her own blood at our feet? Yao Lu was sinking in a world of pain so great, she could not afford the liberating luxury of crying. She feared her own emotions; she repressed them and dissociated them in an effort to avoid feeling the beating pain.

I began pointing it out, inviting her to recognize it as it was caught in the grotesque image before us. A few minutes later, out of the powerful silence that marked her split-off emotions, the floodgates began to open and the long pent-up despair began to pour out from behind her impenetrable walls of stone:

> I have no future.

6.1.4 Prognostics of abuse as a mirror to reality

The end of her third trimester was nearing for Yao Lu. The relationship with her mother was again taken over by a new conflict. Fears about going into labor emerged, and Yao Lu remained uncertain about what she wanted to do with her child once he was born. She was bottling up her emotions and unstable. The idea of adoption was additionally destabilizing to her. An anxiety hurricane was closing in stealthily and in the midst of its vortex you could make out Marcelo's unrelenting yoke. It was time to take action!

She had been letting me know, in small and courageous ways, some of the details of his way of acting. He never left without first getting what he wanted. He would hide from us, control our girl, or send us messages to show off his power framed by or on her body. Certain that it was coming, I predicted the next likely episode of abuse and I communicated it to Yao Lu. I told her he would make her feel forced to do something against her will, and that she should think about it when it was happening. Thus, she might be better able to retrace her emotional state, to recognize what emotions she might be eluding, so that she might use them more consciously to inform her actions. I was attempting to shed some light into the hazy confusion, to *reinforce her ego functions*, in an attempt to help her construct an observing and supportive self. I felt my paternalism was necessary. I had to protect her from the imminent hazards and dangers in her life, and to guide her through the darkness.

I tried to make explicit the implicitly embedded messages Marcelo sent her. I highlighted her his bluntness and dryness, the emotional violence that nearly extinguished her, the intimidation, and his in-exhaustible desire to dominate her sexually by exploiting her in-securities. I emphasized the imperative of fighting for *her happiness*, in lieu of abdicating to that of the other, and of not giving up. I suggested she think about her dilemma around adoption too. We would accompany her; her conflicted dream of being a mother was arriving a few years early.

Yao Lu was not quite ready, so we would also have to protect a baby who, although her child, should not be an object to be "owned", and he needed his safety, rights, and well-being to be protected too. She asked me if children looked more like their fathers or their mothers. I imagined she was anguished by the possibility of a con-stant reminder of another abusing man. But that was my own reading of her question. Our girl shied away from her Chinese identity too![5]

In time, and after another one of my adventures in search of Yao Lu in the darkest corners of Madrid, a few other marginal guys from the street would tell me that the father of the baby was a North African, now imprisoned for a violent crime that was explained to me as a payback. Yao Lu never mentioned it. I don't know if she even knew; some of her experiences remained inaccessible. They were buried deep within. Or maybe our girl did know after all, and they were kept firmly hidden.

Soon enough, Marcelo reappeared on the scene. Yao Lu was once again vulnerable to his domineering, to his invasion and contempt, to his psychological abuse, wrapped in promises and smooth words. But there was more clarity by then. She remembered our reading between the lines of his email messages. She remembered the conclusions we reached and what she needed to try to learn. Our girl remembered how days before, he had wanted to go to the secluded far end of a park. She said no at the time, that that was it, and demanded that he give her back her belongings. Apparently he snickered at her, shortly thereafter asking her contemptuously for a kiss.

> I remembered what you said, about him not letting me dress the way I wanted, but how he then undressed me, without my consent. That hurt, but it was true and I knew that you were telling me for my own good.

Our girl thought it through, she kept our discussion in mind, and she walked away from him, determined. She let me know later, that she felt tremendously overwhelmed by Marcelo, that she couldn't think, even when he was not present, and that at times, *suicide* seemed a viable *option*. She explained how he was critical towards her mother, while over the phone he would sweet-talk her. In anger, she told me how Marcelo had asked her if she had had sexual relations with me, but using of a much cruder term. Irritated, she let me know, both sure and unsure of herself at once, that I was her educator, and that that would not be appropriate nor respectful! *What a new and positive view of a relationship that was automatically negatively (or at best ambivalently) charged at the beginning, given my status, due to my gender, as a potential abuser. She was beginning to feel secure, calm in her relationship with me.* Yao Lu wanted to remain firm in her commitment; she asked that our conversations continue.

> The thing is, that I want to talk, because otherwise, I'm all alone [...] I am going to prove to everyone that I can do things. If he doesn't take my words seriously [in reference to Marcelo] then I'll show him with my... hmm... activit...
>   Do you mean acts or Actions?
>   Yea, actions.

It would still take us a while to free our girl from the clutches of this individual, who persevered in nightly calls, calls that became explicitly degrading and humiliating when she showed herself to be strong, and veered towards sarcastic contemptuousness when she showed herself more vulnerable or closer to him. What a mixed blessing new technology can be. Having her cell phone all night was a commodity that contributed to keeping her trapped.

But when I felt it could help her, I suggested we do a web search together to unmask the thief of innocence. I got an emphatic yes from Yao Lu, and after exploring the corners of the Web, the moment was punctuated by the following comment:

> I think I will be able to deal with my problem with guys. I'm going to tell my psychiatrist.

But abuse is crystallized in psychic dependence and our enemy still managed to see her for a few more days, terrorizing her and making her flee into her inner world. She stayed with him, living as a ghost, terrorized and split off, without daring to separate from him completely, for in doing so endless fears and insecurities would resurface. Conversely, by remaining submitted and tied to him, she was seduced by the illusion of being protected from her primary fears of abandonment.

The fog, however, had begun to thin out and although she may not have had enough strength when facing him, I did. And the day came when we ran into each other, face to face, walking along the sidewalk.

6.1.5 Constricting guilt and separation anxieties

«All in due time», I would tell Yao Lu, and maybe we should first take a detour in these pages to better understand what was in play in my encounter with Marcelo; how Yao Lu's process had unfolded, and what kept her stuck.

Her pregnancy had come to full term, and Yao Lu gave birth to a healthy and beautiful baby. She soon started to discover that motherhood required her being bonded to the needs of the dependent and defenseless new being that was her son.

My job also changed. I was now not only walking alongside our girl, but also her infant, who accompanied us in his stroller along cafeteria terraces, plazas, and parks. Truth be told, we were now accompanying him; we had to be attentive to his needs and protect him, soothe his anxieties with our presence. My attention had to be very diversified in these times.

There were days when Yao Lu seemed to feel very happy with this considerable addition to her world. She was in love with her child and in spite of her own attachment difficulties, she cradled and rocked him, serenading him with a singsong of whispers. The new mother was learning fast. She showed me how to give him a bottle as she had been taught, how to cradle his frail little head in the safety of a graceful movement. I encouraged her to speak to him, and showed her how her son reflexively held onto her fingers tightly with his minuscule hands. It was his way of making sure his mommy would not go anywhere. He needed her! As I demonstrated this, I spoke to him and moved my hands in a synchronized interaction with the rhythm of the baby's movements. It seemed to be a dance. Yao Lu chuckled and participated in curiosity while we laid the groundwork for her baby to form a subjective state of his own.[6]

She invited me to hold the baby one day and he started to cry—a good sign. He became anxious when separated from her and I rapidly returned him to Yao Lu, who then soothed him with soft murmurs and rocking caresses.

This phase was one of considerable complexity. I had to support our girl without undermining her emerging and fragile self-esteem as a mother. At the same time, I tried to tactfully point out the necessary care she had to provide her child. He was her son, but he was at risk of emotional deprivation as she unconsciously tried to tend to her own needs. But how to blame her for it? She had so many![7]

I accompanied her in the discovery of motherhood, a simultaneously fearful and hopeful one, encouraging her to freely explore that longed-for bond. Nevertheless, our girl's anxieties were everpresent, and she frequently found it difficult to connect and meet all of her baby's needs. Amidst nervous laughter, one day she told me that maybe I could be the one to look after him!

I suggested then that we calmly speak of the issue that had been sidestepped. First, I was an educator of boys, girls, girl-mothers, and even babies... but *I could not look after and take charge of her son*. We had to face the feared dilemma, ever present in the minds of us all and so difficult to speak of, of adoption or another form of foster care. I validated how difficult it must be for her. Handing over her child, grown and nurtured inside her for nine months, was bound to be painful even to think about, and more painful perhaps for her, an adoptive daughter who still had the injury of rejection and abandonment by her primary figures. Adoption and abandonment were the heads and tails of the same reality (Múgica, 2006). They came into play in her emotional world and, needless to say, in her capacity to make a decision.

A few days later, as we were already expecting, the first symptoms of her budding internal crisis began to surface. Our girl wanted to go outside, carrying her baby in the sweltering heat of August in Madrid. She was unable to connect with the needs and vulnerabilities of her son, whom she unwittingly objectified, turning him into a mere companion. The baby was absorbed into Yao Lu's own needs, instead of retaining a healthy separateness. Her son gradually ceased demanding the soothing echo of his anxieties in the maternal relationship, and began turning into a baby that was too good and too silent (Bion, 1990; Miller, 1981).[8]

He needed more care than she was able to provide, and I—and all the professionals involved in this case—did not seem to be able to support her and compensate for the deficits they both faced.

Yao Lu's paranoid defenses heightened yet again as her mistrust grew, and she felt attacked by those in the maternity home who were there to support her. As part of the necessary protective care of her baby, they would not let her go outside whenever she wanted to. She became irate. In her conversations with me, she verbally attacked them with a long string of insults and expletives. She blurted out that I was on their side. Overwhelmed and in tears, she claimed that we were only looking to help her son and not her, that we had abandoned her, *that we loved him more!* She did not and could not see that we were all working to support her, particularly given how her role as a mother was embedded in the injurious deficits of her own childhood.

In this paranoid crisis, where we had all turned into villains, I invited her to make sure she was correct, reminding her to pay close attention to the slightest detail, lest we do something to help her and it passed undetected. It would truly be catastrophic to miss out on the very help she was demanding if it were offered. In that hypervigilant context, I pointed out some academic books that I had brought, following a request of hers.

I managed to loosen the grip of that skewed and pathological view of her situation that afternoon. I accompanied and also confronted her, soft and subtle. Held as we were by our strengthened bond, her paranoia did not become consolidated into anger, but uncertainty and silly grins emerged instead. Calmness returned and her tears of frustration were replaced by laughter and smiles. Voided of her aggressive and persecutory view, her environment was experienced as welcoming again. Yao Lu's postpartum was proving to be a time of worrisome vulnerabilities and instabilities.

We found ourselves in a similar predicament a few days later. She was going on and on about how she lived in a prison, though I could see that in this *prison* the doors always remained open. Working like this was not always easy. I was also functioning in the context of a residential setting for single mothers and some of the mothers there, understandably, did not help me whatsoever in the work with Yao Lu. They looked at me with suspicion, and invited Yao Lu to have doubts about us and about me in particular. Men were often vilified. Why would they not be? Many of those women were right. After ending up pregnant, they had been abandoned.

I constantly found myself walking on a tightrope of judgments and prejudices that made me very alert to whatever I said and did so as to not be misinterpreted. I needed to be accepted and *used* as another source of support, gradually, within a multidisciplinary team, as I worked in very diverse and shifting contexts. Yao Lu had a few problematic friendships and as would happen to any teenager in her situation, they influenced her views. «This is a prison!» she exclaimed anxiously. As the suggestive innocent inquirer that I was, I got onboard with the view of imprisonment in a residential facility for single mothers with an open door policy, acting as if she might in fact be right. As I accompanied her, I thought out loud that in any event, it would just be the ground floor that was a prison because, it was the only one with bars on the windows! I shrugged my shoulders in humor and murmured, as if I were on my own, that maybe it was to prevent burglars from coming in, and not to impede girls from exiting through the windows because there was a door... and it was open![9]

Our girl began to smile, making her way out of a paranoid haze. I made the most of it and slightly raised my voice, as one does when surprised, pointing out that barred windows could be seen on the houses around us... «There are captives everywhere!». Yao Lu was in stitches. *We could not have been working here for so many months and not notice such a numerous population of convicts!* She kept on laughing. With her amusement that afternoon, her anxieties facing the complexities of motherhood began to lift again. Instead of responding with an attack, she continued to laugh.

We spoke of the strengths and fragilities of babies that afternoon, and of the imperative to meet their affective needs. Since they were influenced and vulnerable to everything, it was important to protect them from many dangers. Yao Lu listened and agreed that, if it was so suggested in the maternity home, she would accept not going out with the baby in the midday heat. Then her feelings started to emerge. She explained that she was bored, sad, and lonely and that she felt vulnerable to everything and anything. She was finding it hard to devote herself to the demands of parenting this tiny other, as influenced as she was by the emptiness of her own needs.

I was getting ready to leave on a much-needed vacation to hike along the mountain crests of Picos de Europa.[10] Despite erratic cell phone reception, I agreed to call her, so that she could feel my support even from faraway places. Her fears of abandonment would hopefully not break in as they insistently knocked at her door with Soledad at their side. Yao Lu had to keep the path of words open; it was through these conversations that we managed to keep that enemy of ours at bay. Our girl needed to stay in touch with me as a secure tie. In a way, maybe I did too, so I could stay calm despite the distance, remain connected, and not worry too much.

Two weeks later, after I returned from my vacation, she confessed that she felt overwhelmed and flooded by feelings of guilt that hindered her even more in her maternal functions, from which she wished and urgently needed to unbind herself.

Being a mother is really hard, Javier.

Distraught, she felt the need to flee and also started to freeze with uncertainty before her child. He, instead of externalizing his anxieties with frequent or unrelenting cries, slept more and more. Her paranoid crises were on the rise and so was my stress; I felt I had to calm things down and take care of both of them. I felt torn and divided. I felt alternatively angry, happy, sad, and I longed to distance myself from my inner conflict. This was probably similar to what was likely going on for Yao Lu, with the constant risk of affective dysregulation. I did not dissociate as she did—at least not as a common and established answer to my own states of affective hyperarousal,—but I did feel battered in the choppy seas of all those emotions, as if I were in a tsunami. I attempted to regulate my feelings and at the same time regulate our intersubjective space. Hence my stress! In my experience with Yao Lu, there were times when I ended up feeling dazed, scattered, tired, and almost paralyzed in the emotional tsunami we had to work and maneuver in. I frequently woke up in the thick of her non-symbolized communication, trying to re-settle myself in the middle of it all so I could continue working (Bromberg, 1996, 2003, 2008). I was pseudo-dissociated!

She could be disdainful and demanding. Some days she managed to connect with her child, but others, she became more leery, and she even had a hard time looking at him. She told me that she was afraid of his deep and penetrating gaze. Instead of sitting him towards her on her lap—eyes meeting eyes—she placed him looking out, as she glanced at him sideways, fearful of the feelings that could surface.

She would ask me to purchase things, and even give her money. Everything she would ask for, she demanded inappropriately, in rage and tears. *Saying good-bye was scary and somehow, this young girl-mother of ours picked up on it and felt she was going to have to say good-bye soon.* One day she threatened to prostitute herself because of us, claiming that she was not getting any help.

She entered into an emotionally manipulative and exploitative game of threats, where I was set up as the victimizer. If I gave in, I would lose whatever power and respect I had earned in the relationship as a *therapeutic educator*, allowing her to control the relationship according to her impulsive and fluctuating emotions, and allowing her to be controlled by them as well. Yao Lu toyed with the other, reflecting the seriousness of her past injuries and of the present situation. The times were tough.

She started to get back to the maternity home late, and although those who worked there tried to set reasonable limits and curfews, you could feel the buildup of frustration on their end. These tensions began to spill over onto me, in the form of incomprehensible conflicts with the maternity home staff, or at least I interpreted them that way. I absorbed the conflicts and attempted to circumvent the staff diplomatically. Both for my team and myself, getting into arguments about competencies or professional methods made little sense. I understood that Yao Lu was able to push expert workers to their wits' end. I worked for Yao Lu, and we all wanted to be able to contribute to the main and common goal, the maintenance of her stability. It was no easy task.

On *an emotionally stormy day* they let me know that our girl had settled down and had gone up to her room and seemed calm, staring into space and quiet. I tried, in a gentle and conciliatory way, to suggest that perhaps the opposite was true and that we needed to be very alert. In her mind, she may have already been galloping towards a dangerous course.

Her outbursts came and went in abrupt temperamental whirlwinds, and the strains and responsibilities of motherhood, as well as the fears of an uncertain future, were projected out in anger, often against me: «Don't look at my child!», or «Don't use his name!»— «Ok, Yao Lu, I won't use his name»—«Don't use mine either!» ... And just as suddenly as the outbursts had arrived, they simmered down in slightly bashful smiles the next day, in search of forgiveness. It was then that new windows opened, through which we could calmly speak about the preceding crises and the repair of the damage.

But tranquil moments did not last long. These were times of extreme instability. I feared for Yao Lu, and for the wellbeing of her son. I had my own insecurities as I worked in multiple contexts, some in which I did not feel welcomed, let alone supported. Every day was a mystery. I knew *there were concerns about how many of these arduous tasks and difficult experiences I could handle.* My job was to accompany her and to protect our connection. I had to work from this healing relationship of ours, to avoid doing harm, and to guarantee the safety of a mother, child, and myself as well.

6.1.6 Relational dynamics of abuse and the oscillating maternal relationship

Soledad had kept up the onslaught. Fear and insecurity kept Yao Lu subjugated to the ghosts of her past, which she found in the relationship with Marcelo, that she still maintained as an illusory salve.

The persistent tensions between her mother and herself continued. Through the fissures in their relationship, our stealthy enemy Soledad slipped in, escorted by Marcelo and an entire army of fears. Yao Lu told me that at night, when the world seemed to calm down and settle into sleep, she would find herself embroiled in grisly battles with this undesirable companion who came to visit her. Lonely Yao Lu, though surrounded by others, wanted to have friends her age, and the arrival of her son seemed to increase that absence. She felt both trapped in and at the same time alienated from her emotions, and others as well—both alienated and intruded upon as her anxieties surged.

Her mother, unable to tolerate her own anxieties and concerns as she faced her daughter's problems, tended to dump them on her in the form of guilt-inducing and re-victimizing reprimands. Instead of feeling maternal support to face her trembling fears, Yao Lu felt her own anxieties increase, in a constant feeling of impending disaster. She doubted whether she was loved or not. In the grips of *that* fear, she acted out angrily towards her mother in never-ending disputes, constantly putting their love to the test. From the animosity and maternal reprimands, which she actively seemed to bring about, she found the confirmation that she was unlovable and deserved to be rejected.[11]

Moreover, Yao Lu's mother felt her daughter did not love her, and she would accuse her of it, which wreaked emotional havoc. She frequently felt hurt by her daughter's angry outbursts and *acting out*, but she also helped generate these outbursts herself in the midst of volleying of reciprocating anxieties, therefore participating in the fulfillment of Yao Lu's negative omens about their relationship. Anxiety generated anxiety and, both being wrapped up in it, they remained trapped in the mutuality of their conflict. Nevertheless, drop-by-drop, step-by-step, they would gradually manage to improve.

Both were stuck in an entanglement of reprimands, anger, and guilt that bound them tightly together in conflict, yet kept them distant from their sad feelings, which they lived through alone and in fear. They each reactively dumped their anxiety onto the other who, far from being able to resolve them, returned them in a pathological and all-encompassing spiral.

Yao Lu's mother, a prisoner of her own restlessness, tended to point out Yao Lu's flaws, and thus chained her to past failures. Then how was she to build on her past? Are new houses constructed with worm-infested beams?

It was necessary to build with new and firm pillars, but where could these be "found"? The anxiety made sense, but it was massive. Yao Lu's painful experiences and torments also highlighted the narcissistic aspects of an adoptive mother.

One day, Yao Lu confronted me in anger:

> Do you think I go with guys to offer them my body?
>
> Who told you that? [Not answering her question, but redirecting it towards another, for it was obvious that the question was part of a narrative different from mine.]
>
> My mother used to tell me before all the time: You just go to get fondled!

Her mother, without being aware of it, kept her chained to an identity ingrained in the world-view we were precisely trying to de-construct. She kept her bound to that part of herself who submitted to men. Mother and daughter were ensnared by their own fears, each of them reaching the limits of their tolerance for one another, but at the same time connected by the power of their love, of their affection, and by the history they shared.

Marcelo, and Soledad, propelled Yao Lu to find ways to dissociate the threats and anxiety they themselves produced in her, and to some extent they took over her will. They attempted to get our girl to "put one of the oldest coping strategies to elude fear into practice: sub-mission" (Marina, 2006).[12] How terrible and yet how common! How "normal" it is to live subjugated and prey to one's fears, to endure and survive, in lieu of courageously fighting to find a way out of one's torments and of constructing something new! Courage is a scarce value, for it easily disappears in favor of comfort and the avoidance of fear. Nonetheless, Yao Lu was brave, and she communicated through struggle in cryptic and intriguing paradoxes.

Faced with the breakdown of verbal communication, silence began to be not just a form of withdrawal but also a means of communica-tion. Through the silence she conveyed her anxiety and pain. But this silence also activated anxieties in her mother, who dumped them on Yao Lu, and so increased those of our girl. Neither of them received soothing reassurance from the other. So these anxieties, remained active and fermented in the obscure echo of their inner worlds, emerging overnight. Yao Lu had nightmares in which her mother and herself fought violently. Our girl did not feel free to open up to her. The blanket of unease surrounding them grew, so our girl reverted to her pained communicative silence, at which point her mother would default to more reprimands.

There were days when Yao Lu did want to talk, in contrast to her emotional obscurantism. She would be waiting for my arrival, or blaming me if I were not punctual, with an amused smile, «Don't be late!!». She tapped her wrist with her index finger, arching her eyebrows with healthy humor. I had frequently waited for her for hours, or had many a time searched for her down streets and plazas, alert and worried, burdened with my fears. I held my tongue.

The mother's hurtful messages about our girl's identity as a woman produced precisely the attitudes of rebelliousness and frustration that seemed to push her closer to the perverse proposals of Marcelo. Her mother, prey to her own anxieties, had hurled at her on more than one occasion, «you're a slut!». Yao Lu reacted either by completely withdrawing or by acting out the message itself, and defiantly confirming her mother's dire prognosis, or by exploding in dramatic anger. All of these alternatives refueled the problematic dynamic between the two.

As to her relation to Marcelo, I saw Yao Lu as sad and defeated before him, though wishing to be able to extricate herself from the ceaseless harassment. My posture varied: at times I had to act as an educator, a mentor, a father; at others as a mother or, simply, as a silent companion walking by her side. Yao Lu was stuck in a relationship that plunged her into despair and bound her to false security. In her relationship with the other—with the evil and powerful other—it seemed to me that there was actually a part of her identity that was lost in (or to) him. After all, there had always been varying degrees of submission to men in her life, and breaking away produced intense fear not just of losing him, but part of who she was as well.

When I came across that individual on the sidewalk, face to face, recognizing him from the online picture, I had to control my fears and my wrath. I knew that if he was capable of showing up at the residential setting for young mothers to harass our girl as she had described it to me, he would be capable of many things. I also knew that if he manipulated his way to see Yao Lu, it would be because she was once again emotionally trapped. How unfair and cruel! Our girl had already returned his dodgy and deceitful gifts, brave and resilient even in her unsteadiness—She had dumped him! This was new; she had done so herself, in person. Having always been used and then rejected, this was a major achievement! Days prior, when I had asked her about her feelings following this great victory, she glowed as she said: «Proud».

What was this guy doing here then? He went right on by me, our shoulders almost brushing up against each other on the sidewalk. I approached the guard that morning and asked if that individual was looking for Yao Lu. I had doubts whether it was him; since I had never seen him before. But it was. He had told the guard that he had spoken with Yao Lu's mother, who was sick, and they had agreed he would stop by to pick her up. In a happy play of circumstances, that day her mother was actually speaking with her inside the maternity home and he was not let in. Such danger!

Apparently, the subject had been posting threatening signs around the area. I was on my way back from taking a walk, killing time, and *reflecting* on the situation while our girl went on speaking with her mother inside. My intuition said that she may have hoped for my arrival to interrupt them, but I considered it more fitting that she speak with her mother at the time.

As the staff explained how the events had taken place I spotted a sign with a picture of Yao Lu with a list of degrading comments pinned to a tree trunk, and the extent of this individual's scheming, and the danger he posed, suddenly became clear to me. I ripped it down. Everything fell into place now. Infuriated, I called our director. Together we decided I would file a police report myself if Yao Lu was unable to do so, that I should speak about it with them and then go with both of them, mother and daughter, to the police station. It was on the morning of a Saturday.

Given the clear risks that these events brought to light, I worriedly went to see the daughter, mother, and the new baby. I first had to stop Yao Lu, who ran into the street to meet me, her precarious stability shattered, overflowing with fear. When I informed them of the situation, she replied that she suspected it, that she knew it in fact, that the guy had already threatened her with blackmail in every sphere of her life if she left him. Together we agreed to go to the police station, and mother and daughter were joined in precarious mutual support. I did not show them the sign until we got to the precinct. I did not want to trigger a three-generation maternal-filial crisis in the street.

Yao Lu trusted me and, despite feeling agitated, she managed to keep it together. Her mother was not faring as well though; she commenced guilt-tripping her daughter, insisting that she already knew that this was a bad man, that she had told her and had warned her about it. Of course, she was overlooking the fact that she had herself been duped by this impostor's sugarcoated and deceitful words over the phone! She had even come to tell Yao Lu on one occasion that our girl should listen to him, because he seemed to be a good guy. What a mess! She obviously had not known about everything else, and the maltreatment, which our girl, in her anxious secrecy, was incapable of talking about to her mother.

Yao Lu's agitation, lead me to be very directive to contain her mother's anxieties. If I were unsuccessful, it would be a catastrophe. I encouraged our girl to get her ID from her bedroom, and while she did so, I stayed with Mom assessing, soothing, and redirecting her anxieties, not to mention my own! I had just brushed past the malefactor, shoulder to shoulder. My anger towards him and the situation, was still visceral. I listened to my feelings in order to be able to be supportive, to redirect the tension, and continue working from a place of dispassionate reason as much as possible.

I spoke quickly with her mother. She also needed someone to hold and contain her, but she and her daughter were not in a session for therapeutic family work with our psychiatrist. We were unexpectedly in the open of the street. It was difficult and produced tension in all of us.

Shortly thereafter we were facing the doors to the police station. While her mother parked, I showed Yao Lu the sign, asking her not to tear it up before handing it over to her, because we would need to show it to the police. As she held herself together, she anxiously burst into tears and asked for her mother not to go in with her, because she would «have a heart attack». I would go in. A few minutes later, her mother joined us and the three of us were in a room, Yao Lu sobbing inconsolably; her mother, in a display of her tough-love strength, told her «Don't cry... Hey, why are you crying?», drying her tears with affection, but from a distance.

Without being fully aware of it, the mother asked Yao Lu once again to distance herself and ignore her feelings, instead of attending to them. I explained that Yao Lu, her daughter, had many reasons to cry and perhaps this was precisely the time she needed to do so. I pointed this out as gently and tactfully as I could, yet the abyss between them was clear. Her Mother's anxiety slipped right out anyways, in a new guilt-inducing comment that in reality was stemming from her wish to be supportive, «Yao Lu, let's see if this serves as a lesson to you so it doesn't happen again». Discrete, present, silent, I watched them.

I tried to redefine the situation and to redirect them supportively so that Marcelo would not sneak in between them. I pointed out how positive it was for them to be able to be there together, loving each other and being supportive of each other in such a difficult moment. I looked at our girl's mother as I spoke, and could see tears welling up. After all of this, profoundly moved, she told me how thankful she was to all of us. For me, that morning was thanks enough.

The time for our statement arrived. I identified myself to the police as a therapeutic-educator, and explained Yao Lu's atypical situation. We were both led into another room. *Her statement was jarring, intensely so, the most gruesome I had ever had to hear. That was one of the reasons why it was such an effort to write all of this down, and why it has been so hard again now, to sit and read over my notes for the sake of conveying it here.*

We remained there for close to three hours. With me by her side, Yao Lu told a nice female police officer how she had come in contact with Marcelo and about the first time they met shortly after she got to the maternity home at age sixteen. She told her how he took her to a dark storage room where he raped her multiple times, grabbing her by the neck. She spoke of other things he did to her and of the pain he inflicted, and an endless list of details that would only highlight the darkest and most atrocious side of that human being.

Yao Lu, perhaps picking up on the shock of this police officer, said as if to take care of her:

I just have problems, you know? That's why we go to therapy and all ... I'm working on it to get better ...

Throughout her entire statement, Yao Lu did not shed a single tear. On several occasions, I was under the impression the police officer questioning her was about to cry herself. Re-experiencing the trauma would be too painful, so in order to tell her story, she had to reel it off without emotion in an unbroken chain of words. But it seemed to offer hope despite the overwhelming sorrow it evoked. These were firm, and decisive steps for Yao Lu's future; or so I thought.

The next morning I returned to the police station on my own, armed with a file that included Marcelo's demographic information, a history of shady transactions on the Internet, as well as his address and photograph. It was the result of the research that I had done.

They were surprised and enormously thankful, because as they said, it was a thorough investigation and it made their job easier. I had the feeling, nevertheless, that this individual was an old acquaintance of the police. Right there before me, they took off after a rapid succession of phone calls and messages in code. In less than 45 minutes, our enemy and companion to Soledad was under arrest. Our girl could breathe, and so could I. Marcelo was in police custody and they would keep him overnight.

I finished providing my statement, handed over the documents and, as I mentally read over them, I was flooded by my emotions that I contained with visible effort. The police officers thanked me for my involvement and said, «Hardly anybody does this». With a quiver in my voice, which was hard to conceal—absurd even to try at this point—and tears in my eyes, my heart spoke these clarifying words:

> She's my little girl, you see.

I was her therapeutic educator, but I felt like an anguished father, shaken up by the experiences of his violated daughter. I had sought to take care of her wherever she might have been, sometimes managing to do so and other times unable to find her; always trying to accompany and not to intrude, in our goal of helping her develop her freedom and autonomy.

I was only there temporarily, to help her defeat the unrelenting hurricane of her torments, for this, my—our—hurt little girl.

Notes

1 A. Slade (2006), in her reflective parenting programs, refers to this as *facilitating wondering*, and notes the importance of an imaginative wondering full of open possibilities, in which the recognition, interest, and curious exploration by the parents—and there is a parallel with educators—of the child's experiences, as well as considering them separate from their own, helps children validate their own separate experiences in a protected space where they can develop in freedom and autonomy.

   This method, applied to our adolescent, validated Yao Lu's experience and, more importantly, liberated her from mine, at a time when I had worriedly been looking for her. It allowed for her to distance herself from me, without making her responsible for my own anxieties, and thus recognizing what was hers, mine, and ours. It fostered mentalization (Fonagy & Target, 2006) without inducing her to adapt to me in a kind of imposed bond referred to by A. Miller (1981).

2 I am referring not just to children but also to the adult educator who frequently forgets he or she was once also a child and that back then the world was seen through a different lens. Perhaps what is ideal in a job like this is to be able to navigate between both worlds.

3 It must be noted that in the original version in Spanish, Loneliness (Soledad), (which might also be translated as solitude but would then lack the isolating pain of loneliness) is a common woman's name; and hence the narrative assumes the use of the feminine "her", when speaking of the externalized and literarily personified noun Loneliness. Translation runs the risk of losing linguistic and cultural nuances. Unfortunately, the ambivalent poetry encapsulated in culturally specific words may be one of them. For a more extended view on narrative externalization, the reader is invited to look into p.63 in *Narrative Means to Therapeutic Ends*, by White and Epston.

4 In addition to this, and granted that all communication has both report (content) and command (relational expectation) aspects (Watzlawick et al., 2011), in the content of Marcelo's communication there was a demand for submission, as is understood by Ghent (1990).

5 In the letters received by Xinran, her book *Message from an unknown Chinese mother* (2010) documents parallel processes of identity rejection, which could be understood as adaptive dissociations of adoptees to the new cultural and linguistic environment, as well as an effort at integrating themselves and expelling parts of their *self*. It is possible that these parts are recalled in the memories and ruptures of an origin that was neither warm nor welcoming.

6 Research by J. Jaffe et al. (2001), *Rhythms and dialogues in infancy*, reflects the importance of matching between the caretaker/mother and the unfolding of affect regulation in a non-causal but co-regulated and co-constructed interaction. Their research, which is based on the idea of mutual regulation in the vocal and rhythmic matching of the adult with the child, and the child with the adult, points out that it is not perfect coordination of child and adult that predicts a

secure attachment, but the midrange of bidirectional coordination. The extremes result in disorganized attachment with excessive matching) and avoidant attachment (with insufficient matching).

Fonagy & Target (2006), referencing Gergely & Watson (1996) and their article «The social biofeedback model of parent affect mirroring»—*International Journal of Psycho-Analysis,* 77, 1181–1212—describe how it is precisely in that world of imperfect interpersonal contingencies of the caretaker, where the baby can start to differentiate its different self-states, along a process of *social biofeedback* with the other. It is during those moments of rupture and repair in the me-you relationship, of empathic and congruent contingencies with the internal state of the child, as well as the marking of the difference of those affective states of the other—mine and yours—without precluding their existence and recognition, where a secure attachment would be forged (Fonagy & Target, 2006). Applying all of this to our work, a complete empathic fusion with Yao Lu, was not only impossible, but not desirable. The relational space between us, allowing us to explore possible points of connection and frustrating "meconnaissances", also allowed for a "mutual surrender" (Ghent, 1990) in a space of "thirdness" (Benjamin, 2004)—was where our relationship could create something new, just as she could now do with her child.

7   D. N. Stern (1995) described the motherhood constellation as a convergence of evocative experiences and discourses that get activated in the mother, which reorganize and affirm her identity. They happen both inside an outside, and are born out of her relationship with her own mother, and her mother's relationship to her as a child, as well as her own relationship as a mother to her baby (p.172). Yao Lu had interacted with many caretaking figures in her life, so whom would she do this with, and how? with her adoptive mother? her birth mother? through transferences with her psychiatrist? Yao Lu's lived experiences were certainly echoing and shifting, especially in her role as a mother to her child, and her interactions with him stirred up many feelings. Would she feel good enough? Would she think about whether he loved her? And of special significance for her: would she feel lovable?

This special relationship, as can be intuited, required a great deal of mental effort of our girl and, as Green (1980) suggested, Yao Lu found it very hard to tolerate her child's developmentally appropriate needs just like other mothers with histories of abandonment by their own mothers, or who had not grown up with reliable caretakers, because she was stirred up by her own history of unmet needs. And in her inability to think of her child's immaturity and dependency, and the dissociation of her own painful experience of the past, she pushed her baby into being 'independent', in ways that were well beyond what he could do, so that the latter, perhaps in her fantasy, would take care of her (p.99). Would Yao Lu be able to reorganize her identity and modify the different parts of her self, to devote herself to a motherhood that was «good enough»?

8   Just as described by Bion (1990), he was turning into a baby adapted to the mother, through the splitting off of his own anxieties, which were no longer

tolerated by her. Alice Miller (1981) spoke about this as a cathexis of the baby by the narcissistic injury of the mother, through the suppression of its emotional needs to cover those latent in her.

9   To go into Yao Lu's world like this allowed for its questioning from the inside, as an ally who could then be able to step out and still be there by her side. There was an alliance emerging akin to what Ringstrom (2007) described, bidirectional intersubjective, that moved us from a predominant one-way intersubjectivity where I was empathic and could connect with what she felt, to a two-way intersubjectivity where *we* knew what *we* felt, or at least could have a sense of it. It took us both past the limitations of our respective personality structures (p.69). We were forging what others have called an *implicit relational knowing* (Lyons-Ruth et al., 1998). In the playful space created between us, in that humorous moment of meeting of ours, she could question, filter, and perhaps modify the possibility of her future experiences with men as less constricting.

10   Picos de Europa National Park is a mountain range in the north of Spain with rocky peaks, sinuous mountain trails and spectacular views.

11   These types of relational dynamics are characteristic of some families with adopted children who develop difficulties in belonging to their new family, which frequently has become a family precisely with their own arrival. Neuburger (1997) believes that «the adoptive child will generally feel more strongly towards biological aspects, notwithstanding, or perhaps due to, the parental denial of them. At that point, the child will thus only be left with trying to prove the fairness of his or her view, namely: that he or she is not loved as a biological child, but for the capacity to please the adoptive parents. In order to do this, the child will put the alleged parental love to the test with ever increasing provocations. Once the limit to the parents' tolerance is met, the child will feel the hypothesis of not being truly loved confirmed. Revenge will be the only thing left!» *Translation is from the text in Spanish and my own. The original, which does not yet seem to be translated into English to this author's knowledge, is published in French under: Neuburger, R. (1995) «Le mythe familial» ESF, Paris.*

12   Marina (2006) «*Anatomía del Miedo: Un Tratado Sobre la Valentía*» *(The Anatomy of Fear: A Treatise on Courage)*—Author's translation.

Chapter 7

Autumn: Crisis as danger and opportunity

7.1 Times of crises and the dilemmas of adoption-foster care

7.1.1 Acting out as a means of separation and the risks of prostitution

It was a sad time. Our "workplace" had been changing. Yao Lu said she was bored and that she missed our conversations. With Autumn on its way, the climate was not favorable for strolling around with a baby and the inside of cafés was choked by harmful tobacco smoke (smoking in public venues was still allowed then). In spite of this, there were days we managed to converse under the sun, on some pleasant terrace as we used to, and she would then speak nostalgically of our times past, lost amidst the turmoil of anxieties and changes of the present, as her eyes teemed with tears that delicately slid down as she spoke.

The thought of having to separate from her son saddened her. She feared losing his love, and that he would no longer recognize her after a few years. She felt forced to face the loss of the most significant bond—she said—perhaps of her life. They would not lose touch altogether because she retained visitation. The importance of their relationship had to be balanced with their right to be protected, even if it was from one another.

Keeping mother and child together would have been giving in to a biologically based bias, privileging Yao Lu's immediate needs, to the detriment of her baby, who, although loved, would not have his needs and rights adequately or sufficiently met (Barudy & Dantagnan, 2005).

DOI: 10.4324/9781003261490-7

She was also beginning to come to terms with her own shortcomings and limitations as a parent. She let me know what being a mother was like for her, her expression turning sad. And she sighed:

> I'm not ready... to be a good mother.

She spoke of the hardships of waking up at all hours, of the lack of sleep, of being a parent too young, of having a serious problem with men to work on. Our hurt girl, breaking down after acting out, full of invisible anxieties, wanted to improve and better herself, to rise above her deep sorrows, to move forward and succeed with our support to hold her. What a heavy burden of daily difficulties! What a great need for help and support to face such early and serious deficits.

As the paralyzing fear relaxed its grip on the safety of our attachment relationship, Yao Lu allowed herself to speak about the difficulties of motherhood, and about her anxieties as she faced a new and painful separation that was now understood as necessary for both of them. In a new moment, she connected with the depths of her pain and let me know how profoundly she feared the farewell. How could she not? With a life story like hers!

Yao Lu wished for her son to have a happy childhood, different from her own. But her mother, a grandmother at the time, unable to comprehend Yao Lu's difficulties, also feared the loss of her grandson. So once again, she laid all responsibility onto her daughter and guilt-tripped her by insisting that if she were to give the child up for foster care, he would soon forget her and she would be doomed to the loss of his love.

This was a very unfortunate and harmful message, for it not only emotionally alienated Yao Lu from her son, but it also robbed her of any positive feelings or closeness (even if only in fantasy) with her biological mother and her family of origin, and thus reinforced her inner compartmentalization and divided *self.*

To hand her child over to foster care reactivated all her fears of abandonment; it turned her into an *abandoning mother* in the eyes of her own adoptive mother, who herself had threatened to leave her on so many occasions because of her problematic behavior. Tensions were running high and another great storm swiftly arrived.

As I was arriving at the maternity home one day I just about tripped over Yao Lu as she angrily stormed out, fiercely slamming the door behind her. Shocked, I looked back towards her, and then at the caseworkers who had urgently called out for the door to be unlatched. They were about to give me an explanation, but there was no time and off I ran after her. *She was leaving without her son*, dressed in flashy, tight-fitting clothes, wrapped up in belts, bracelets, and gaudy trinkets.

A great crisis had arrived. The risk was extreme. Somehow, she had gotten wind of the imminent foster placement from an indiscreet comment by an exasperated maternity home staff. Even though it was explicitly part of the work in her therapy, she experienced the comment as punitive, as a reprimand. It inflicted unbearable pain on our young mother, and she was acting out self-destructively. She was rushing off to prostitute herself.

In the thick of this emotional tempest, she warned me that it was no time for me to be there, that since "Madrid" was going to take her child, *she was off to find a new pregnancy* «I'm going to do whatever I want!». Oh the risks, I thought, and I tried to calm her down. The possibility of a bitter separation without a goodbye was swiftly becoming a reality. I did not know how she found out, but I presumed that the news was thrown at her abruptly and insensitively in a moment of frustration. This undermined our therapeutic goals of making her increasingly aware of what was at stake and of making her feel part of this decision. We were also trying to support her in the painful process of saying «see you soon» to her baby—not goodbye—to be able to continue working through her difficulties while he lived under the care of a generous family. Something had not been conveyed properly. I had a feeling it had partly to do with the paranoid projections of our girl, which at the same time generated insecurities in the team of professionals.

I walked hastily at her side, within the forcefield of her exploding anger; I encouraged her to think of her child. For brief moments she reconnected; but then amidst screams and wild gesticulations she yelled out at me: «I don't want you to come! My boyfriend doesn't like educators around, because you always report my boyfriends!». Did our girl have a boyfriend again? By then I had already become the target of the stares of numerous pedestrians. I was deeply fearful for her. In her anger, unmoored, she was decidedly getting closer to the subway tracks and the train was making its way into the station. Our nerves were running high: we held our ground. I took a deep breath when the moments of danger came, remaining close enough to grab her if she teetered on those stiletto heels, yet far enough away that I would not provoke her.

The doors of the train car opened and in she went like a gust of wind to the opposite end. I gave her space—what was I to do? Back in her residential setting, they had hastily opened the door for her, possibly fearful of her explosive rage. They had not been too considerate in their dealings with me either. Even though they knew me and were at least partially aware of my work with her, at times the staff had dismissively treated me as if I were one of their client's maltreating males. But I do not want to divert too much attention to the difficulties I faced with institutional relations. Never until then had Yao Lu needed me to physically restrain or grab her. But what was I to do now? How could I get her to go back to the maternity home?

I felt like a branch broken off from our team, cast adrift in a no-man's land of highly charged yet ridiculous conflicts of interest and power that such a case brought to the fore. Wanting to promote Yao Lu's progress, how could we take on risks while lessening hers? Someone in power had to step in, I thought nervously. This type of work required child protective services to be at once coherent, efficient, and flexible. It was just wrong that I was finding myself in a situation like this where magnified perhaps by my own anxiety, I was drowning in organizational rivalries that in no way helped a girl like Yao Lu, and made my task much more difficult. I called our director. She calmly reassured me and gave me a few pointers on how to deal with our adolescent, as she assumed responsibility for the mediation with the professionals outside our team. I quickly recovered my balance.

Yao Lu was weaving through the crowd in a jam-packed subway station during rush hour. I followed her, lost her, saw her, and lost her again, and then caught a glimpse of her once more as she disappeared at the top of a crowded escalator. As I rapidly made my way up, excusing myself repeatedly, I came across the furtive and elusive glance of the man who, in the recent past, had told her *that she was in need of a man*, reiterating that he loved her and then chucked her aside. He was on his way down the adjacent steps. He recognized me. I must have been a well-known person among certain sectors of the marginal underworld like this individual. Down I went after him. Our girl was not upstairs, and they had both vanished by then. Yao Lu had probably alerted him of my presence.

During the next few hours, I searched for her ceaselessly, but as time ticked by, I gradually lost hope and made my way back to the maternity home. Now they did invite me in! I said I would rather wait outside, having a cup of coffee just in case she appeared, and would they please give me a call if she did. But she did not return.

7.1.2 Crisis and hospital setting interventions

I did not manage to speak with Yao Lu until the following day. She would not tell me where she was, but she did answer the phone when she saw my number and did not hang up. She was falling apart and told me she was giving up, because she would never get to be happy. I took it as a despairing plea for help. She had spent the night out, surrounded by questionable individuals and many dangers, and by now she knew that she had likely precipitated the separation from her child. He was already in protective care, and in response to her great loss she was throwing herself into unprotected and risky situations.

I suggested we meet to talk in a place known to both of us. I was worried about her and wanted to convey that. I assured her I would be waiting, regardless of her decision over the phone, so she could have time to think. She did not show up, nonetheless I waited. I made up my mind to send her a text message letting her know that I was where I said I would be, and I assured her that I was not giving up and neither should she. She was to keep fighting!

The next time I was able to see her, she was an inpatient in the adolescent psychiatry ward of a hospital in Madrid.

i   *Self-destruction as a defense*

She shared her pain with me when she saw me. Simply put, she had grown tired of trying and was surrendering to torments, thus protecting herself from disappointed hopes and the fear of failure.[1]

> Javier, you see... I was born to suffer.

I was accompanying her in a situation new to me too, in the adolescent psychiatry ward of a hospital. We were surrounded and observed by the staff, who kept a watchful eye over everyone. Some children spoke with family members, others remained silent. Others were without visitors yet and paced nervously, as if powered by inexhaustible batteries.

Never before had I been in a psychiatric hospital, and these circumstances were stressful to say the least for a first time. It was a short tearful visit. With the loss of our bearings and fears closing in, the ground seemed to crumble under our feet; Yao Lu was captive in her fortress of fears. The light of hope had to be turned on once again.

Immersed in crisis, Yao Lu was exposing herself to great risks. If she would allow herself to connect with her pain, instead of fleeing and protecting herself in dissociation, perhaps she could finally come out from her torments. I had to offer myself as a crutch to lean on. How is one to reconstruct oneself if everything is unstable? I had to give her the security she needed to be able to have faith. These were potential moments of holding, mourning, and recovery, while she was temporarily under the watchful eye of a hospital setting. A new opportunity needed to take shape, so that she would no longer be hiding in fear and dissociation.

She spoke to me of the man in the prior encounter, not a new boyfriend as she had snapped at me in the subway, but something else. She spoke of her continuing confusion about the differences between love and sex, and of a terrible feeling after each and every one of her relations. She had spent the night in a shabby hostel, only to be abandoned. She also explained that she had met another young man and that he seemed good, though she always found some flaw in *the good ones* and cast them aside, always remaining with *the bad ones*, the abusing ones. It was not a fully conscious pattern, but it seemed to be coming into her awareness, and it was terrifying.

She was again lost, yet a small ray of hope peeked into the darkness of her world. Following her brief hospital stay, *the doors to her Home in our Therapeutic Community opened up for her once again (her child was now no longer with her, and she was still a teenage-girl in much need of accompaniment and therapeutic work).* *She wanted to go back!* Throughout the entire time she was living at the facility for young mothers, some of her old educators from our therapeutic community had kept in contact with her in one form or other. Some would go with her to her doctor appointments in the mornings, or to the psychotherapy sessions with our director; others had gone to visit her when she gave birth to her baby. The relationships with the professionals from our Home had remained alive. Yao Lu was a beloved girl, despite the difficulties she generated and it was important that she feel loved.

Once she was doing better, we were able to go take a short walk in one of the nearby parks. She launched an attack, but it was feeble. Trembling, she said we made her suffer. Her words were neither forceful nor heartfelt, but loaded with sorrow for the loss of her son, which she still seemed to not completely comprehend. I was gentle yet firm in my invitation to reflect. Trying to maintain my stance of emotional containment, I tried to allow the underlying sadness to express itself. We spoke of her relations with men, of the feeling of guilt she had after being with each and every one of them, of how she initiated contacts without wanting to go to bed, but generally ending up doing so. Yao Lu said how she had suffered and never been happy her whole life, and in a breaking voice, she also said she felt that if she had not been abused in China, her problems here would not exist.

This was hard to hear, since our girl's words came from the depths of her soul. The tears began to spill and soaked her clothes. I was only looking to be supportive so she could identify the feelings, so the time came to gently close up the spring I had tapped into. I did not want to open up old injuries without being certain of my ability to close them back up. After all, I too was still learning.

I allowed her to pull herself back together, and reaching for some light humor, I announced that I had forgotten to give her a present that she might possibly like. As if it were a small treasure, I presented her in a reverential gesture with a gift that could have been fit for royalty, handing over a new pack of paper tissues that I fished out of my pocket. She smiled, and as she took the tissues, the overflowing tears started to dry, her smile grew big, and a small chuckle of tear-drenched laughter slipped out.

We had both worked very hard to create therapeutic places outside the conventional setting, such as a city park busy with people milling around us. The time to go back to the hospital had come and, feeling protected in our space, she let me in on a little secret:

> You know I think a lot... and even though it might seem like I'm not thinking, I think all day long...

Had she felt held? Had I managed to accompany her along her turbulent experiences? Right before I left the adolescent ward, my day livened up:

> Thanks for coming Javier ... I needed it.
>   You're welcome, Yao Lu.

It had been tough for us both, but her words had made that arduous day worthwhile.

ii. *What does a good father do?*

When I visited Yao Lu in the hospital again the day after she had blamed me for her loss, I had a clearer idea of where our talking should happen. She needed a culprit in order to articulate the pain. In blaming others, she avoided taking on responsibility for her own decisions and for the consequences of her actions. While her life was anchored in very early injuries, we wanted to help her develop the capability to lead her present life in a balanced and autonomous way. From her position as a victim, she frequently became the victimizer of those who were trying to support her, and sometimes of her self too.

I guided her to a bench facing a nearby playground. After calmly listening to her pain I invited her to go deeper into her feeling. Tentative tears began gliding down her cheeks. Then the dam cracked. They were gushing, soaking her pants, her hands. At times, with her head hanging low, the tears even seemed to jump right over her glasses.

Her sadness was profound and the sobs were with us for a long while. She spoke of the love for her son; of her wish to be with him; of the possibility of kneeling and pleading before whomever she had to, for his return. I listened. Her son seemed to be the center of her life, but she had put him in clear and serious danger. Yao Lu counted the days since she had seen him last and said she would take her life. Without him, she was worthless; she would go back out onto the street, which was the only thing she did feel good at. Victim to her grieving and torments, she was becoming her own aggressor.

I listened and helped her calm down, redirecting her feeling of deep pain. Yao Lu loved her son and she wanted to love him, but she did not quite know how. We spoke of her ending her life, but we also spoke of the alternatives opening up before her, leading her towards a less difficult, healthier path. We spoke of the team of educators she knew well, whom she could lean on when she went back to the Home. Calmness started to appear, stemming the flow of tears, which began rolling down more peacefully. They dried, disappeared, and resurfaced more softly now. From her son she could receive strength to fight and not give up, but first she was to understand herself, work through the probable loss of her child, and to achieve a more mature perspective towards him than that of an "object" she owned.

> I'm going to ask you a question Javier: Why have they taken my son?

I took a deep breath, prudently trying to avoid both the landmines of a too complex and of a too simple answer. Her son had been neglected, poorly stimulated, and put into situations with grave risks, for example when she surrounded herself with men who abused her. I helped her think through answers that could be found in each of the examples.

We were sitting facing each other on a bench in El Retiro, a marvelous, classic park in Madrid. The play area before us had been slowly filling up with children and parents, trickling in with each of Yao Lu's saddened tears. Gently, I suggested that we face the playground, where the world of early childhood was now twirling. Close by, just a few meters away, over a dozen boys and girls, with mothers and fathers, played and interacted spontaneously. Some parents helped their children with walking, others gestured exaggeratedly as only parents do, enthralled in the emotional and imaginary world of

their children. Children cried, laughed, swung, or explored. I invited
her to contemplate the view, and waited in silence.

We were watching a different reality, the longed-for world of
childhood; we were attentive observers, both distant and very near.
Our girl began to open her eyes to a new quotidian and foreign life.
We were temporary guests in this world, and its inhabitants opened it
up for us through their games. Suddenly, with loud crackling
laughter, a smiling girl of about four appeared between some shrubs.
She was followed by her little brother who approached us with
wobbly steps, his small arms outstretched and his eyes full of wonder.
I pointed them out and together we contemplated the spectacle. Their
father, crouching down low and moving with giant-like steps, was
immersed in that tiny imaginary forest where they seemed to lose
themselves in their play as they looked in awe around them. He
seemed to rediscover the world through their eyes and through their
thousand questions. Other parents pushed their children on swings. I
encouraged her to look closely, to let herself feel, to *listen to herself
feel*, while I remained by her side in caring silence.

Yao Lu did look closely, and with the dampening of her eyes I
sensed the dawning of a new light. The strings of her heart got tugged
on as she watched the laughing children. I asked what feelings she
could see there,

> There's love and... accompaniment...

From our observation post, she had been able to catch a glimpse of
parenting that her history, pain, and anger, had kept away from her.
The picture was full of love, yes, and of accompaniment. The parents
accompanied their children in exploring the world, trying to look at it
through their eyes, to understand it as children do. Moreover, those
parents who were able to allow this, like the father who took giant
steps in an imaginary forest, would likely rediscover the world
through their children, who then magically, could become «companions» to their parents, thus constructing a life they could share.

Reflecting on this picture, Yao Lu stated that, in her recent and
turbulent urban wanderings, her son had accompanied her more than
she had been able to for him. She seemed to be beginning to

understand her difficulty. I encouraged her to gather her strength. Although her son was no longer with her, she had a valuable reason to fight. We would not give up. We would continue together, accompanying her on her path.

A few days later she returned to our Home, where a new task awaited us both. Each change in location involved small yet significant relational readjustments for us. We had been through so many experiences already! As an educator, I was known in the Therapeutic Community Home. I had worked there a few years earlier, prior to my hiatus to go abroad a few weeks after Yao Lu's arrival. Many of the educators and some of the children were known to me. I had worked with a few of them there. We all had questions, but the need to maintain the hard-earned confidentiality did not allow me to respond to many of them. I had to take care of our girl during this new phase. We were no longer at the maternity home. I imagine Yao Lu had contradictory and ambivalent feelings as she saw me in an environment where other children, to whom I had been an educator before, threw themselves at me for hugs in front of her. Yet Yao Lu still needed my exclusive attention, and the protection of our unique relationship.

Our first day working in the Home was one of few words and mutual observation, as if our relationship of accompaniment were beginning anew. It was a new setting for the two of us. Our history had changed us, yet I let her know when we went out for a walk, that I was concerned about her seeming *too well*. It was as if she needed to please everyone. She told me that she was fed up with doing everything right, but that didn't match her behavior. She went back to her dissociated world, with radiant smiles on the outside, but wanting to cry on the inside. We wondered if the sadness would surface upon seeing her son soon. In fact, we were certain it would. Within days, our girl disappeared again, and ended up admitted into the hospital psychiatric ward.

iii. *The eternal companions*

I did not know in what state I would find Yao Lu. Two educators had stumbled upon her in the subway, and were witness to how, in a violent and aggressive frenzy, she bit a policeman and ended up admitted. She was falling apart. She smiled when she saw me. Despite the staff on the unit assuring her I would come, she insisted that nobody would visit.

Many days had passed since our conversation when our girl said she was at the end of her rope and could go on no longer. She smiled, and distanced herself from her feelings. She told me about her wandering around the city and about her dangerous dance with prostitution. At the time I decided against delving into those unsavory details, which would emerge later.

As I churned inside, I became interested in unlocking her "happy face" dissociation that we called «appearance». If I were to have come across Yao Lu on the street and not known her story, I would have undoubtedly believed her to be a happy girl! She was quite the theatrical prodigy, enchanting and charming, yet false and unstable. As she began to speak, she leaned back in her chair as if gaining distance from her words. I inquired into the underlying feelings, attempting to pass over the harrowing details of her prostitution. I concentrated on her effusive non-verbal meta-communication, which I thought was tied to her dissociation.[2] I attempted to minimize the distance between her narrative and her elusive *split-off self*, reflecting on the pain she must feel—a pain that was so great, that in order to tell her story, she had to protect herself behind ample smiles. I reminded her of my impression when I sensed everything was going «too well», and she recognized her usual defense of hiding by displaying a mask of smiles to everyone else, an important part of her highly changeable *false self*.

This girl needed to *listen to her feelings*, for the happiness she sought could only be found in an inner life that included her pain as well. I pointed at her heart, and asked how she was feeling, trying to provide a unifying thread amongst her multiple self experience and the emotional world she hid inside.

> I'm a mess.

I invited her to be as honest as she could. Her story echoed with pain between the smiles. She began to associate, instead of escaping into alienated states. Our girl-mother began to let her head hang low, as she met her forgotten tears. Her expression turned sad and somber, closer and truer to her emotions. Despair ruled. According to her interpretation of her life, the explanation was a simple one: she had grown tired of waiting for something good to happen. She did not want to prostitute herself; she wanted to be with her child, and her mother, and she was at a loss as how to do so. She felt like giving up, she smiled, she cried, or both at the same time. I reminded her that pretending was unnecessary, that I was there for her however she felt inside.

Amidst this teary outpour, she looked for the watch on my wrist. I asked if she wanted me to leave for the day, and she emphatically gestured «No!». Slowly, she got herself up to go find something she wanted to show me, a few more tears trickled down, and our hospital visiting hours ran out. Yao Lu seemed on the edge of an abyss; on one hand wanting to let go, and on the other, hoping to find the strength to fight her way out. I left sad and moved by the despair exuding from my hurt little girl, yet with a warm glow inside me. When I said goodbye, without expecting anything, she looked out from her sorrows and thanked me for the time we shared.

> Talking has really helped.

Her sorrows had lightened, just like the burden of my own, although I found it unavoidable to carry a few away with me.

She spent several days in the hospital, at times blocking off her feelings, and at others spilling out in a spring of tears, so much so that I wondered if she could become dehydrated. The psychiatric nurses and staff would ask me how I thought she was doing, puzzled over such abundant weeping. Except for the rare occasion, our girl did not allow others to see even a hint of her sadness. With patience, she gradually regained the shelter of the containment of our relationship, even in that hospital setting. She began again to associate with her emotions, courageously allowing herself to express her sadness. I would leave emotionally drained.

We must have been quite the confusing spectacle through the glass walls of the visitors' room. I would find a girl, all smiles, who after a short conversation, would break down and cry in a calm constant stream of tears. She would lean forwards resting her head on the table between us, and we would then speak of her suppressed sorrows. I always left reflecting on her progress, and on what to work on next, on my experiences and intuitions, which I routinely shared with our director and psychiatrist through email. I wondered if I had pushed her too far or too little, but I always stayed prudent. My motto was always: *better fall short than push her too much.*

One day I found her with a huge smile, while at the same time telling me that she no longer knew how to go on (as paradoxical a communication as it gets!) and that she had made up her mind to be a teenager. More than being just a teenager, it came across as unbridled and harmful turmoil. I reflected on the appropriateness of her wanting to be an adolescent, because she was. «And a mother too!», she added. Exactly! How to reconcile them both? We explored the intrinsic nature of each one of those conditions, and began to play over the table, as I staged the dilemma with my hands. «Adolescent» for her meant going out, parties, and studying; and I stuck out the thumb, index, and middle fingers of my left hand and placed them in a pyramid raising my hand above them on the table, as I repeated her words: «going out, parties, studying». I asked about that mother issue of hers. What was that all about? «To take care of» and «to accompany» emerged, and I added «to love», also pointing them out with the same fingers on my right hand.

Our girl felt she was one more than the other some days, and she struggled with how to reconcile them. Yet she presented as exorbitantly happy! I pointed out that for her adolescence was about: «Parties, going out, studying!». Rhythmically moving my bouncing left hand in a triangular motion on the table. «Parties, going out, studying! I'm a teenager!». Followed by being a mother. «To take care of, to accompany, to love!». My right hand then rhythmically danced around on the table too. «To take care of, accompany, to love! Party, go out!», until one hand would crash into the other and both collapsed—«I give up!». My tensely entangled hands tried to raise themselves up again unsuccessfully, whilst I said «Teenager, party, mother!» and then they collapsed yet again. Indeed, reconciling the two identities must have been difficult.

Maybe it was about learning how to walk again, neither exclusively as an adolescent nor exclusively as a mother, but in the integration of both, without either of them erasing the other. She was in need of guidance on how not only to reconstruct herself, but also on how to understand herself. She was moved by my staging of her present dilemma and leaned over her arm on the table, allowing a small lock of hair to fall over the tears in her eyes. Her caged anxiety slipped out.

> How do I go about it?

We had already spoken a great deal about her problematic relationship with men. To do so again would perhaps be stifling now; and our teenager was living with the burden and pressure of a companion far more powerful than those men. Yao Lu was followed by *Soledad!* We took a deeper look at *that relationship*.

When could Soledad have appeared for the first time? «In China... when my father was abusive». And thus we began narrating a new story of her life. She was followed all the way from China, by a detached yet highly present invisible companion who flew beside her on the airplane. I played it out visually, our girl flying in the airplane of my right hand in a slow arc over the table, as the flapping and silent "Loneliness" of my left hand followed.

> I've always thought of committing suicide, since I was little; but I never did... because it's not a good life.

That was precisely evidence of her resilience. Yao Lu was a fighter. In bravely shoving aside this perennial companion, she had been leaning on another inconspicuous traveler in her life. Who would that be?

Throughout her long and arduous journey, and despite all her hardships, Yao Lu also had a companion called *"Esperanza"* (*Hope*), and this powerful ally helped by casting rays of light in her times of torment. Hope encouraged her to survive her heartaches; it opened windows and doors to her emotional fortress, allowing in a refreshing breeze that chased away *Soledad* and filled Yao Lu with new dreams, in the face of her life's despair. *Esperanza* was that light in the dark tunnel.

Sadness caught up with Yao Lu in that story. Her expression changed dramatically before me, from a flirtatious adolescent, to become that of a somber adolescent-maturing-mother; a girl still, but more in tune with her desperate emotional state, yet illuminated by the power of renewed *Hope*.

Notes

1 This could be understood as a form of "submssion" in Ghent's (1990) terminology, a submission to replace the more genuine and longed-for "surrender" to another, since Yao Lu, in letting herself go and giving-in to the misfortunes of her predicament, she liberated herself, or at least gave herself the illusion, from an existence of torture and difficult emotions. It diminished the anxiety produced by feeling temporarily, or partially, in control of the reigns of her life. In this way, she freed herself. In relinquishing the fight and her resilience, she managed to create an illusion of freedom and expansion-of-self in her, to slide towards the external world without feeling her internal conflict. In her decision, the price was to submit.
2 Through the metacommunication we followed a thread that allowed us to track the dissociated self-parts, to find them—even to work with them—observing and talking about her different self-states, as Bromberg (1996) might say. There were times I even positioned myself as an auxiliary-ego who would be able to include her alienated states and thus help her regain her agency, still diluted in her submission to men.

Chapter 8

Winter: Silent speech

8.1 Appearances of a different nature: The surrogate family

The return to the Home was difficult. For Yao Lu it involved a step back on her path, now not just hers but also ours. Once again, nuances emerged in our relational space. Surrounded by a Home of smiles, anger, sobs, and tears, but above all accompanied by the sparkles of Hope, we created new conversational spaces.

The first day, I let her guide me along places infused with her positive memories. As I walked alongside her, she reminisced. It was a nice journey, far from the bustle and noise of our city. Our neighborhood now was a green and calm area. That morning she surrounded us with her memories. I accompanied her on her nostalgic voyage, taking imaginary snapshots. We passed by bus stops that took her back to her adoptive mother. We walked past the racks of teenage magazines at a newsstand. And we stopped unexpectedly to breathe in deeply the essences of a flower shop, for the first time. We were back, yet also in a new place.

8.1.1 A context of multiple relationships

For Yao Lu, being separated from her child heightened her anxieties and increased her instability. Going back to a setting with children, like the group Home, had its benefits, but it also involved risks. Where else could she go? We all knew her here and could continue to work with her. There would be no need to open up to strangers again, with all the added anxieties that this would entail. Nonetheless, I could feel that her

DOI: 10.4324/9781003261490-8

unconscious fears and emotional turmoil were occasionally pushing her, shutting her down. She communicated in the opacity of smiling silences. I had to be alert, to interpret, and to meta-communicate, so as to weave these silences together and provide a link to the lost parts of her self.

During my weekly visits to the Home, we worked in a world with little privacy. Though the other children and educators tried not to bother us, there were regular interruptions. The setting was open and communal and, as in a family, as in life itself, we found ourselves surrounded by this teeming micro-world. The scene highlighted Yao Lu's behavior when she sat drawn into herself, or when she raised her voice to be heard, or when she took cover under protective smiles when bright tears flowed only moments before. It all gave me a sharper picture to work with.

Carefully, I commented on her different ways of relating to me, which were influenced by the presence of whomever else was around, or just passing by. I invited her to reflect on her relationship with me, and indirectly with herself, and to think about how to remain centered while surrounded by others. We moved deeper into her world, and deeper into my own. I also tried to remain centered and aware of my emotions.

As I gradually stopped obsessing over trying to understand her better, I began looking at the accompaniment as a mutual journey of self-discovery. If she invited me on her process— it was really ours by now— I would welcome getting to know her more. We were accompanying each other, and in doing so, we were meeting each other too. My goal was to help Yao Lu to listen to herself feel, without running away, but I had to be able to do that too. The task was to navigate in the rough seas of her tormented memories, and to come back safely to shore.

8.1.2 Calling for lost innocence

Communicating with Yao Lu suddenly became more complex. Hidden behind a curtain of dissociative smiles, she would regularly say «everything is fine». One of those days I invited her to explain how she felt, and eventually she began revealing her fears. I saw that talking about her feelings and experiences was terrifying, and we returned to the issue of prostitution that I had previously decided to set aside. She did not want to end up a prostitute, but believed it to be an easy path. She knew it would involve further distance from her child and her mother, both of whom she loved. As a prostitute she split away from herself, trapped in a fierce emotional drama, desensitized yet a prisoner within.

To open herself to her feelings about her mother and her child would expose her to the losses and mourning she was bound to find. Yao Lu was trapped. She had long walked at the edge of the abyss of disconnection on one side, and of despair on the other. She had to be pointed in the right direction to regain Hope, or she would become a prisoner to herself, the most onerous slavery as Seneca once wrote. For Yao Lu, prostitution was a choice that would enslave her to the fears she was trying to escape.

She began to tell me she wanted to change, that she wanted *to be* well and to enjoy her family's company. She longed for a family she had never had. Tethered as she was to the memories of past abuse in China, it seemed a very unlikely dream. I suggested we speak of the faraway land. She remembered her father as an abusive tormenter. She also remembered a caretaker in the orphanage—who, following Yao Lu's courageous escape from home, continued to traumatize her, now sexually, holding her to silence with cruel threats.

After our many experiences together, I could recognize the range of emotions festering behind her smiles. We knew each other well enough at this point so that I knew how far we could go and still contain her emotions. She was investing her trust in me, sharing her feelings when she could.

We approached a bench in the park and I suggested that, with my support, she claim something back. I invited her to imagine that she had the opportunity to tell that evil caretaker what she felt and what she wanted him to acknowledge. I reminded her that I was right there firmly by her side, supporting her with my hand on her shoulder. Her feelings began to emerge from behind superficial smiles. Yao Lu told him to leave her alone, that he had turned her adolescence into a tyranny that had not allowed her to enjoy her life. He had stolen her childhood and she wanted it back. Together we would reclaim it. We would send that ever so present tormenting ghost that lived in her *traumatic memory*, to hell. That was enough.

I felt that to remain there, facing the bench, would be too revictimizing, after exposing her to a pain she had yet to work through.

As we kept on talking we walked to another bench, creating a distance from the previous moment. Yao Lu's distancing smiles were gone. She could have been a part of the *Guernica*.[1] Her facial expression contracted and froze as she let her wailing pain flow outwards. The picture was far from pretty. It moved me deeply to see her in such a state. I imagine it was something like a father whose daughter's pain was his as well. I am not a father, but what a powerful relationship it must be! Surrounded by my caring, her voice breaking, she spoke tentatively. She spoke of being afraid, of not knowing how to be without a man; of feeling insecure without one; concluding that she threw herself at men who treated her badly because she was unable to find herself without them. In essence, Yao Lu felt she did not know how *to be* without the presence of the *other* as a man. She did not want to have that feeling. She was recognizing what the nature of her relationships with men was for the first time, spontaneously. She was exploring her feelings, threading together her disconnected worlds, sustained as she was by the trust of our accompaniment. This way of relating is what I refer to as the *implicit dance of covert meanings*, the aura of which I had felt the day we met. There it was in plain sight, now recognized by our brave girl. I could hardly believe her growing capacity for *insight*, and the effort she made to become self-aware. I accompanied her in the beautiful journey of a girl meeting her lost self. As she spoke, her words flowed as freely as her tears.

When Yao Lu was not in a relationship with somebody, I could feel more acutely the subtle teetering of the foundations of an identity vulnerable to crumbling. It was as if there was a part of her that she sought out within the enmeshed relationships with abusive men. I would feel, when those men were not around, how she adapted and molded to me, in a subtle and flirtatious search for a safe refuge, oscillating unconsciously between *submission* and *surrender*. Somehow, being in those relationships, being close and distant from her feelings protected her from disintegration. With other men, she would likely automatically become submissive, thus putting them in control of her.[2] I was very aware of these patterns of behaviors and wanted to help her see them, but only when she was ready. That moment was approaching, and with her *insights*, she was taking the lead herself.

It was important to support that controlled emotional "break-down". By holding her feelings so she could thus regain her balance, by looking into her past experiences in the presence of a supportive and caretaking male figure, "breakdown" would be her defensive armor, not her self.

Our girl had no wish for the other's pity. She wanted to overcome the difficulties, to be strong, get better, and make up for the time lost. Those were her words. She was resilient, even if she dissociated much of the pain she had to deal with. And if she picked up on other people's pity, she had to resist the lure of continuing to be a victim. What she perceived from them could become a powerful trap. How was she to rebuild new relationships and a new self-image, if what she felt from others was that she was damaged and worthless? Yao Lu needed fertile ground to grow on and restructure her narrative. Hopefully, this work would let her build new ones.

Our relationship was situated where it could resist sociocultural pressures that kept in place an identity as a *permanent victim* of past abuse. This would put in place an identity constructed on the foundation of our Hope as the *successful survivor* of the torments and tormentors.

Protected in our team's accompaniment, Yao Lu could begin to vary the scripts and work out new representations of herself. We were working on the development of an alternative narrative to her life, in which Yao Lu was a fighter, a survivor of her troubled origins, who battled Soledad with her faithful companion Hope, as with our team.

Made of a concoction of accompaniment and hope, we were creating the specific and unique balm for her real wounds, something that cannot be commoditized and purchased. This balm belongs only in the context of artisanal care aimed at the individual. Hence the unease and incomprehension when human care is crammed into a model of quantifiable (dosage) commodities (farmaceuticals).

8.1.3 The need for stable maternal care and the fear of abandonment

The mother-daughter relationship was also in turmoil. They distrusted each other, repeatedly putting each other's love and affection to the test. They both feared the loss of affection from the other, keeping the ghost of abandonment alive between them. In a self-fulfilling prophecy, constant arguments became the test of their love. The revisiting of old fears and anger regularly punctuated their meetings.

Her mother, engulfed in the loss of her grandson, prey to anxieties and worry for her daughter, had a very hard time showing support for Yao Lu's brave efforts in trying to change her life, and herself. Quite the opposite, she frequently reminded her that the separation from her son was her own fault, among many others, and this cornered Yao Lu into a deep sense of guilt. This likely had something to do with Yao Lu's mother's own latent feeling of guilt as an adoptive parent. It also made sense that Yao Lu lived in the constant presence of the thought of her absent child, but she also had to live with the unsettling uncertainty about whether her mother was more of a mother to him than her, as if her mother's strident prophecies of oblivion and abandonment were a demonstration of greater love for her grandson. Our girl needed to have a sense of belonging and attachment to something, especially to her family, so she could build a sense of security (Neuburger, 1997).[3]

Unwittingly, her mother constantly reinforced Yao Lu's feelings of abandonment. She had great difficulty in connecting emotionally with her daughter; they were locked in a pattern of mutual distrust and attacks that protected them from feeling their grief; Yet Yao Lu was improving. She began not to return anger as quickly, but listened more reflectively.

It was necessary to recognize the sadness underlying the pain, which both distanced and kept them close, and to search for a new relationship based on their moments of attunement, instead of "dissonant resonance" to use a paradoxical phrase. It was important for them to understand each other, so they could share and continue building a path together.

We spoke of the feelings underlying her mother's comments that echoed throughout Yao Lu's life history and her time with me. The team educators were also faced with holding the mother's anxieties and complaints. She frequently and repeatedly called on the phone. It seemed like a battalion of worries and fears was locked into place in fear of the pain and loss. It spoke to the situation's fragility.

Yao Lu was sad, stirred up by her mother's re-victimizing rants that generated considerable guilt in her. She felt blocked, unable to speak with her mother, and would slide into profound silences. But these silences would unnerve her mother even further. Not receiving any response to her anxieties, she would insist vehemently, pushing her daughter into further silent reclusion that screamed out loud. They fed each other in this mutual dynamic of volleying anxieties, which interestingly enough seemed to parallel Yao Lu's relationships with men, and our girl's submission to the other.

Having been a frequent witness to this type of interaction, such as phone calls that would fade out into a "silent explosion", I invited our girl to calmly put an end to a conversation one day, so we could get to work. When her tears began to flow and there was more warmth in the air, we invited her mother to join us, albeit in imagination, so Yao Lu could tell her then what she had been unable to moments before. We placed a chair in front of ours, and I invited her to imagine her mother seated there, to envision her, and tell her everything she was telling me. And I guaranteed her mother would listen now. She smiled sadly, and began slowly:

> I want you to tell me that you love me, mom. I want you to tell me that I can go back and live with you whenever I want to… that you won't aband … (And she froze for an instant, as if it were too painful to say, while I affectionately lay my hand on her shoulder). That you won't abandon me… I don't want you to tell me of the failures in my past … I want to improve! I don't want to go out on the street!

These were touching moments. Yao Lu needed to feel supported to grow, and I was moved as I listened to this brave girl who put into words everything she had previously been unable to say on the phone.

When she seemed to have finished, we allowed for another long, yet different, silence. I removed the chair, and we affectionately bade her mother farewell with gentle humor. I suggested we go for a walk. This seemed to please her, and without further ado I waited at the door, punctuating the moment and allowing for the important echo of her words, by not diluting them with any of my comments or explanations. She needed to listen to the echo of her feelings and I to mine.

Upon our return, after we said goodbye, I later learned she called up her mother. She was able to tell her that she understood her worry and that she too was afraid, but that she wanted to do things right. Somehow, she was able to convey her need for support, a great little success. Nevertheless, and to my distress, in the weeks that followed mother and daughter did not find a new balance. They had heated arguments, unable to find peace, and Yao Lu fled towards dangerous worlds. Again I would need to turn into a detective to find her and walk back with her on the paths of Hope.

8.1.4 The hidden self

Yao Lu returned from her escapes and runnings-away engulfed in the pain of altogether new wounds. She would then spend days in recovery. As she got better and her smile returned, she would suddenly get hit by the pang of a bad memory or by a word she considered hurtful—from her mother, myself, or any of her peers or educators—and she would again run in terror to her broken identity forged by abuse, sinking in silence into her world of pain. To feel was to suffer, and her tendency was thus to flee into smiling silences, while casting herself into the arms of abusers on the street. In these despairing impulses, the batteries of the horror of her inner world were recharged.

I searched for her with great concern, fearing someday to hear horrific news on television. Some days I reached her through the *messenger chats*, for although I was reluctant to make use of it in the beginning, it was an efficient means to reach our adolescent. I sent out messages suggesting we meet. But it was delicate since I could not see her face for guidance. Nonetheless, although short in her answers, she did not cut off our line of communication. It was not too useful a resource, but it served to tell me that she was still «free» and alive. My concern and fear was that I myself might lose our friend Hope. Another of my worries was that she would become prey to an abuser who would lock her up in the dungeon of his apartment. She had already met a few who could fit the bill.

Subsequent to her returns, I assessed whether to insist on her telling me what happened or not. No, that was not the most important; I could come across like her mother and then... slow down Javier! I was already aware of her horror stories, and my persistence in having her tell me about new ones did not seem to lead to improvement. To keep going down that path, therefore, could be interpreted as a form of intrusion that would unwittingly push her into the abyss of disconnection and the arms of Soledad. Perhaps what was important was to help in her self-exploration and not overwhelm her with my insistence for her to speak, an insistence which would likely stem from my own anxiety as I learned of the perils she was in. My anxieties and concerns when facing the dangers she was in ought not to permeate our shared space for they would push her to clam up in silence. I encouraged her, therefore, to explore the differences and similarities between her *actings out* on the street in retrospective calmness, where she could look at herself with new eyes.

Throughout that period, there was no lack of angry outbursts and, quite frequently, she implicitly invited me into them. Our girl would pour out the rage of her life story over me: she unconsciously invited me to enter her anxiety, so as to be able to explode and dump her undigested pain on me. I was to remain serene.[4] I particularly remember the day when, upon my arrival, I was warned about how angry she was. Taking a deep breath, I left my belongings in the room, and intrigued, went off to explore and take on the new day. She was seated, reading, but her face was the portrait of someone traveling through turbulent worlds, far beyond what was written on that paper. Straightforward, I asked about the degree of her displeasure. «On a one to ten, how much? Or is it more like fifteen?».

«The absolute maximum!», she responded irritated. Calmly, as if it had nothing to do with me, I answered that I also got angry sometimes, but I put on a different face, and showed her mine with slightly baring teeth; a bit comical but in line with the moment. She smiled, but it was gone in a flash. She must have remembered her need to be angry, and went back to her previous appearance. By validating her anger it may have prevented a more uncontrolled confrontation, and by inviting her to assign a numerical value to it, I was inviting her to take ownership of it, making it increasingly hard to project it onto our team. It was the way I found to bring down the heat of the moment too.

I gave her a couple of minutes before we talked, taking them also for myself, so I could gather my wits for a moment that promised to be difficult. Yao Lu's expressions of wrath in moments like these could be understood as her only way of connecting and securing an attachment with the other (albeit hostile), which allowed for her psychic survival (Sonntag, 2007) in the midst of the risk of affective disintegration. From a place of anger, she protected herself with cohesive rage and the clarity of projections.

Immersed in a whirlwind of conflicting experiences as either the doer or the done to (Benjamin, 2004), she made an appeal to the insistence of another educator that it was time to read or study, as if he were the tyrannical ruler of the place, and she told me that if I wanted to talk with her I was to take it up with him. Our girl set us up into many conflicts in ways such as these, unconsciously probing for the team's loopholes while in the presence of other children. Even then, we were all well coordinated. I turned around to ask my colleague, who I was keeping an eye on yet also an ally to, if it was ok for Yao Lu to come with me, trying not to take away authority from the person who was meant to have it at the time. Seconds later, we were marching off, Yao Lu briskly walking full of pride ahead of me, towards our now usual place for conversations.

She began telling me she wanted to be on the street. She felt good there, throwing herself at the first guy who came close; that love at first sight was her thing. The irony was biting; it hid silenced emotions behind the mask of smiles. She unloaded a description of her dangerous misfortunes onto me, in a game that defiantly called for my anxiety. But I remained impassible. I calmly spoke of the street as a rollercoaster, where one could feel the euphoria of the plummet, where heartbeats quickened with the lack of control, where there was excitement, but also a great danger.

The problem was that the street was not a true rollercoaster, it had no rails and did not brake slowly; when it came down, she got hurt. Through her anger, through the smiles, she could not help but communicate, as she did through the metaphorical screams of her behavior, that told us: «Here I am!—Yao Lu—and I have feelings! I'm here, I'm alive... and I feel real bad!». Unconsciously her behavior was the expression of a longing, of a wish, almost a whisper, to be found, to be recognized and seen, even at the risk of appearing quite the opposite.

I concretized her defensive mask of «everything is fine». Weaving it into a tale where she would no longer need it to speak of her tormented inner life, I suggested that perhaps she could begin to slowly remove it and hang it up on one of the hooks on the wall, though it would remain invisible, and it would take time.

The day finally came when I invited her gently to connect with the emotions trapped behind *the transparent mask*. I leaned towards her on the chair, and literally acted as if I were removing the object of dissociation. Affectionately, I untied imaginary knots behind her ears, carefully detaching her invisible mask. She smiled, yet these were not smiles of disconnection. With each knot being untied, tears began sliding out, as a tribute to the sadness she was running from, and she told me:

> This is just the way I am ... I've been like this forever ...

With an abusing and violent father, and a caretaker at an orphanage who intermingled the pretense of care with sexual abuse, blackmail, and neglect, how could she not be like that? What option was left if not hiding for her emotional survival from a world with no outlet? I asked her to *describe the mask*, to make it more visible. «All black, plain, without eyes, no mouth... Dark». It was terrifying, yet liberating, to be able to remove it, however briefly. I invited her to continue down that path of courage. I would stay with her, by her side and if we were in need of a bucket to collect the tears, we would look for one.

Our conversations had inadvertently been condensing themselves into rich forty-five minute sessions. Smiling through her tears, Yao Lu asked me if we could spend what time we had left listening to music and going out for a stroll.

8.1.5 Testing the waters in the fight against Soledad. Counterparadoxes and alter-ego farewells

We had both come a long way in our path together. I was in training—avid to learn, comprehend and find an explanation to each and every one of the experiences we shared, and enormously eager to help and understand her—studying for a master's degree. More than just being a good student, I avidly devoured all the new knowledge. I had to. I had also made notable progress in the way I worked with her, as had she in her self-awareness, introspection, and capacity to symbolize. She now reached into the deeper recesses of her being. Our conversations gave her time to reflect, and they saved her from acting impulsively in flights to or from her dissociated parts. She also began to trust the Home's educators more and looked for their support.

Some days Soledad reappeared and the troubles returned; on others it seemed as if She did not even enter her life. I asked her in amazement how she managed it. It was simple: our girl was learning to make use of fundamental tools, words. When she used them well, she emerged from pathological silences, and was able to come out from behind her usual mask of smiles. Truth be told she was still running serious risks; but her improvements, and the wellbeing secondary to them, as well as her recurrent crises throughout her process, had to be looked at from the perspective that our work had allowed with time. Yao Lu was changing step by step, at moments almost imperceptibly.

I also invited her to be prudent, telling her I was not too sure if now was the right time to take off her invisible mask of smiles and hang it up for good. By doing this, I introduced her to a *counterparadox* that, precisely, gave her strength to do otherwise; and our girl began to talk more and more, where before she would flee in terror.

The surprise came one day when she asked me to go to an Internet café with her and delete the noxious contacts on her *instant messenger*. Sitting before this newly opened window onto the corners of her world, I was stupefied when I saw her email address. It was as if she were introducing me to her alter ego. She used her last names, but a different first name. There, before us, she opened her web of contacts and deleted them one by one. Yao Lu was moved with tears that did not flow, but formed precarious pools at the edge of her eyes; but it was important to help her not feel overwhelmed, to feel sufficiently supported and strong enough to keep moving forward.

The thought of deleting her presence on the internet was coming from her, which was what mattered. Yao Lu began telling me how, years before, she had created that address to contact boys and not be recognized. Her voice, breaking up but still strong, sounded connected, as she explained how, somehow, that alter ego with a different name, was also a part of her.[5]

I invited her to dramatize the moment and in doing so to represent the feelings stirred by her memories. Our girl had mastered the art of communication without speaking. She shivered from head to toe with sadness on her face. It was as if her email address were not hers, but belonged to somebody else, in a parallel world of terrible experiences. Then and there, and in laughter, we spoke a few farewell words.

There, in front of the *webcam*, Yao Lu gave the final click as we said farewell to a secret part of her self, waving our hands together in goodbye. It was a bittersweet moment; although it appeared to be a lighthearted game, the implicit meanings were heavy with pain and confusion. Again, saying goodbye was scary.[6]

Notes

1 In the painting by Picasso (1937), the expression of suffering and horror of the human figure, seizes the viewers' attention.
2 Following the terminology and distinction by Ghent (1990) on submission and surrender.
3 R. Neuburger (1997) refers to a psychic-sense-of-belonging, the «rooting», produced by what he has described as the implanting of the family's myth. When a new member is introduced into the family, by virtue of adoption, this member should be taken-in, comforted, and wrapped-up by a new blanket, with introjects that weave together the member's sense of belonging to that family. However—and this we add ourselves—if the implanting of the family myth is too rigid, it might increase dissociation and rupture in the adoptee's historicity, and in his/her identity. The adoptee would thus experience himself or herself in strongly divided, almost irreconcilable states, as a result of the «traumatic» effects of the loss associated with the new encounter. This likely also has to do with the age of the adoptee at the time of adoption. The older the adoptee, the greater the risk of splitting the self as a way of adapting to the family and their mythology. Or there could be more rebelliousness as a paradoxical test of love and belonging.
4 From the perspective of Eskelinen de Folch (1988), it would be after repeatedly experiencing me as a container who understood her and was not overthrown, working with her with the most intolerable impulses, that Yao Lu could, maybe eventually, make use of me as an internalized object that would strengthen her ego, with increased capacity for reflection, for intuition and verbalization of her own experience. In time, perhaps this would increase her ability to communicate with her internal world, or even recognize it, just as with the external one, in an increasingly tempered and self-regulated way. (Adapted from the author's article T. Eskelinen de Folch (1988), «Communication and containing in child analysis: Towards terminability»).
5 Bromberg (1996) states that there is an important shift, when a part of the self is able to look back on another previously dissociated part of the self, and reflect on it. When a patient's increasing reflective abilities move them from a moment of

dissociation to conflict, they sometimes do not like what they learn about themselves, or what they see (p. 517). He refers to this shift as «standing in the spaces»; that is, to look reflectively upon one's functioning in different circumstances. The achievement of this self-observing capacity allows for a more realistic and fluid awareness of one's selfhood, a "me".

6 This farewell game could be interpreted as my being manipulative, directing her to dissociate a part of her self once again, but it was not so: the petition was coming from, and guided by her. In the dramatization, therefore, we were forging a co-constructed and resilient space for self-discovery, sought by her—a space of transition.

Chapter 9

Spring: Responsibility and freedom

9.1 Angsty freedom

Yao Lu deserved to be free. But how? It was our job to help her take off, but flying is not easy. Yao Lu would get anxious and flee in terror, leaving me once again confused and intrigued. Upon her return, our work would resume, from wherever we had left off, building on and integrating each one of the steps along her path, although on occasion it seemed to be like an acrobatic choreography.

In distancing herself from her past, she was also coming into contact with the very emotions she was fleeing, and she was taken over by anxiety. To feel and to remember terrified her. By running from the fear, she catapulted herself into the street, and so relived her past with men, repeating it through sex rather than remember it. It was her way of dealing with emptiness and pain

Yao Lu had never thought much of herself, as she told me through her tears. She needed us to believe in her in order to build a new life, but to take ownership of her autonomy entailed risk.—She felt the perils acutely. A lifetime of submission to abusive "others" had forged a worthless self, undeserving of anyone's love and affection. Anticipating and avoiding these feelings, instead of confronting them, sent her back to people who tormented her. The improvements in her daily life with constructive external reinforcements were not enough to fill the immense void within. Perhaps a resolution lay in some hidden moment of her past (Miller, 1981). Feeling unworthy of anyone's affection, she was flooded by feelings of worthlessness that

DOI: 10.4324/9781003261490-9

fit a worldview, which had been shaped step by step through her past experiences.

Nonetheless, confronting that universe could give her an opportunity for growth. It was not a matter of 'making' her sad, but of connecting the sadness so as to facilitate the subtle dialogue with her hidden self, concealed behind the fear. She might be brought to tears only to later have access to truer smiles, not the dissociative and distant ones.

Yao Lu sometimes ran from one place to the next, hounded and haunted by her broken feelings. She had to work through these memories and feelings in order to find the strength to forge a new path for her life. And she was doing so. It was surprising. She told me how, when she went out onto the street looking for guys, she did not look for one only, but counted them in tens. She did not quite know why, but she was beginning to try to make sense of it. When, in her misadventures with men, they called her «whore» she said she wouldn't listen, for if she did she would commit suicide.

In the repeated fleeing and reconnecting with her emotions she began to know and to recognize herself, making sense of her relational patterns. Yet she said she simply went to the streets to *avoid* suffering![1]

I frequently contemplated what «being free» might mean for Yao Lu and, specifically, what it might be for her in our relationship of therapeutic accompaniment. Freedom goes beyond just doing whatever one wants, for in freedom lies an intrinsic responsibility. This aspect is however the one that is eluded when we do whatever we please. For Rollo May, freedom involved an individual's agency and growth, and was rooted in being aware of oneself. Without the latter, we would move about the world as instinctual creatures without reflecting on our past, and thus without being able to influence how we might act in the present. (May, 1953, p.160). From this perspective, Yao Lu's freedom, and its increase, resided in her self-awareness. Through the exploration of the nooks and crannies of her fear-filled inner world, and by mastering these fears, she would be able to free herself from them, or find herself in them, and thus transcend, rather than flee them.

In little glimpses, she was getting to know herself more and more, freeing herself from the constricting chains of the past. Maybe then she would be able to have more opportunities for future choice, and from there, to be freer. I told her that, notwithstanding how many times that she ran away, that she *acted out* in her street misadventures, she would continue to be an important person to me and to the whole team. I valued her, and would keep doing so regardless of her relapses. If fear did not let her be free, I would try to awaken in her the courage to believe in her capabilities. I would support her. We had to keep going!

As if she were asking if I were aware of what she had done when she came back from her self-destructive street crises, she would state she had not been at the Home the day of my scheduled visit. It was phrased both as a question and as straightforward statement. In the underlying message, she needed to know if I had worried about her, if she was important to me! Sometimes I had the feeling that her escapades onto the street were public announcements of her intolerable anxiety, her screaming silences.

I thanked her for the diverse ways of trying to communicate with me. I had to pay close attention to gain insight into her emotions, and at times I was slow to catch on, and realized things too late. I hoped that she could understand, and trust, that her feelings, even if they went unexpressed in words, were seen, heard, held, and continued to be important to me, and so could become important for her too, even when she froze and withdrew. After a lifetime of avoiding her emotions, immersing herself in abusive relationships, being transplanted to a new country with a new language, how was she to communicate if not through mimicry, silence, or non-verbal behaviors?

Yao Lu collapsed into tears and laughter, stating she did not know how to communicate if it was not through the disruptive behaviors of her crises. I gradually tried to reflect back to her each one of the challenges she had faced throughout her life, and her improvements. I reflected back a more positive view of herself, to help her apprehend and integrate a new *being* and *becoming* in life. She was going through a rough time and she captured it in two sentences that were as simple as they were complex.[2]

> The thing is, being well stresses me out. I get overwhelmed.

Up until that point, Yao Lu did not usually go out alone because every time she did, her outing ended up in anxiety-ridden escapades full of nocturnal incidents, from which she returned bruised inside and out. She needed to grow her fledgling autonomy. She had to encounter the loneliness of strolling down the sidewalk with herself, and standing tall as she faced her fears, instead of fleeing under their spell.

I was learning to ride a bicycle with my father as a young boy. I pedaled anxiously, but he provided the necessary security by running alongside me, providing balance, both physical and mental. I wished but also feared to find myself alone to face the exhilarating freedom— «Don't let go!». But letting go is necessary, and my father did so many meters before I actually realized it and crashed spectacularly, yet no longer overcome by fear. What a blow! But I had already made progress without *training wheels* and my father, who had sensed that capacity in me *before I had myself,* had confidence in me, and I happily moved forwards and with no help, until I looked! I fell, but by then my balance was, following the brief success, only a matter of practice.

Letting go of Yao Lu was necessary, but only when she could bathe in the confidence of one of her moments of success, because the risks she ran were still too great. Falls are important, for there is a lesson to learn from them, but hers were of a different nature than that of a kid learning how to ride a bike. The faith in her, the trust, was nonetheless basic and necessary, and her dances of resilience could be thought of as training exercises, with reasonable chances of success that she would not falter and fall into overly risky behavior.

I called her on the phone one day, before my visit to the Home. I asked how she was doing. She was happy! Based on her confident tone, I suggested that perhaps given her increasing responsibility, she might meet me at the café terrace we frequently spoke at, instead of my going to pick her up. But I was not sure and wanted to consult with her first. She laughed, and you could sense her excitement over the phone.

—Yes, yes I can! Ok!
—How long do you think it might take you to get ready?
—Five minutes Javier! I'm ready!

She was ready and in less than five minutes, as I waited at the café unsure and trusting at the same time, a girl-mother-teen appeared before me, brimming with an almost child-like delight that she shared with me. There was no holding back the smiles! She was not a baby learning how to walk, nor was she learning to ride a bicycle. She simply appeared, walking. Yet the complexity of it all! Previously, she would run away, full of anxieties and fears, to the torments of the streets, and would return battered days later. This was quite a step toward maturity!

I stood up and proffered the appropriate reverence and salutations required by a prominent figure, yet not making it a mocking or an overly exaggerated act. The truth was that it was an event for both of us, but especially for her. The battle towards freedom was hers, and I was only a companion.

Leaving the Home by herself and going 'in the street', without getting emotionally lost, must have brought mixed feelings, of both hope and fear. I thought through the timing of this, and wondered how to increase the likelihood of its becoming a triumphant moment. To walk under the Spring sun must have produced an exciting euphoria of sorts. For the first time, our girl felt able to keep things under control. In allowing herself that experience, she was sharing her trust with me and making mine grow for her. I thanked her explicitly. What a moment!

Amidst our smiles, her experience of freedom in her inner universe began to shine. After conversing there with me, she happily returned to the Home on her own and as soon as she went in, it slipped right out in earshot of a colleague of mine:

> I'm a grown-up now.

She also began to be more free.

Notes

1 One could establish a link to the research by P. Fonagy and A. Bateman (2008) on borderline patients and their difficulty to think about feelings, because these are frightening! They reactivate a primary *attachment system*, which in Yao Lu could be understood through the lens of her *acting out* and return to abusive situations. Perhaps these abusive situations and their traumatic complexity was a place where she felt «seen» and recognized, in a *true*—and hurting—*self*, in Winnicott's terms,

or at least in one of its parts (Bromberg, 1996), where she could feel more whole in the relationship of submission (Ghent, 1990). What a paradox! Yet what a difficult one to get out of!

2 These sentences were so striking! Her crises would frequently take place after a period of «being well», as she would assure me. We confirmed it and found ways to address her emotional states at the time, using a scale from one to ten to make the assessment easier. Perplexed, I noticed that she was unable to integrate her positive state for long without the dissociated *parts of her self*, which were increasingly distant from her, due to her progressive improvement, from reasserting their influence. Perhaps Yao Lu's predicament could be understood, in a radical reversal of our conventional views, as her having experienced her positive state as alien and frightening, as «not me» (Sullivan, 1953), which she would unconsciously flee for the more familiar, secure and superficially coherent experience of abuse. But, at the same time, she was also beginning to feel the need for a personal change. Through this lens, her *acting out* and other risky behaviors could be understood as security operations (Sullivan, 1953), which sought to mitigate the anxiety of her not-me states, whose tension seemed to increase with each improvement. We understood that these improvements involved the partial loss of old or archaic parts of her *self* which she now found difficult to integrate; and with that dissonance and the increase of anxiety, which our entire active team arduously attempted to help her regulate, her more primary *attachment system* (Fonagy & Bateman, 2008) got reactivated. In that situation, Yao Lu was swept away by the primary figure of the abuser, in whom she could calm the unbearable anxiety in a pseudo-voluntary submission, connected to her primal longing for care and a real connection (Ghent, 1990; Berliner, 1958 in Caflisch, 2012). For a girl dominated by trauma, whose verbal language lacked richness, behavior as a means of communication (Watzlawick et al., 2011) seemed especially relevant. Actions as solution frequently became impulsive in reaction to her affective disintegration. I encouraged her in her progress. How could I not, I was her educator, but I also had to accept her setbacks and not urge her to progress and improve more than she could. Otherwise, I would push her to prematurely distance herself from a part of her (her state as a traumatized and abused girl), which perhaps *I* found difficult to integrate—a not-me of hers for *me* in this case. Without wishing to do so, I could thus maintain the alienation of her early emotional states, in lieu of doing the opposite, which was their integration and our ultimate goal. On these occasions, although it was personally taxing on me, as it was for all of us, we knew that if Yao Lu was going to be able to transcend her abused *self*, and be able to gradually integrate her dissociated parts in a more coherent and less reactive way of being, closer to a *unitary self* (Bromberg, 1996, 2008) and not oscillate in its extremes, we would have to accept those «not-mes'», that moved and jarred us and me profoundly.

Chapter 10

Creating a time of our own: China and Pandora's box

10.1 Chinese culture: An experience beyond the culinary

10.1.1 The taste of China

I had been accompanying Yao Lu for about one year and a half by now. We had shared many experiences. Beginning shortly after we met, and continuing over the course of her pregnancy, we often sat down for a meal together. A pregnant teenager had to eat and, why not at a Chinese restaurant?

At her request, we immersed ourselves with the smells, tastes, and sounds of her past, of her culture. We were surrounded by diners leaning over large bowls, slurping their spicy noodle soups. We could overhear their conversations, the television, or the music. I did not understand a word, and frequently I was the only westerner. The roots of Yao Lu's life came to life for me in these settings.

To the surprise of our girl, who had forgotten her mother tongue, everyone greeted her and tried to speak to her in Chinese, and she had to respond repeatedly: «I don't understand! I'm a Spaniard!». It amused her and she explained: «It's just that "they" do it every time!». We laughed when they brought her a menu with only Chinese characters, unintelligible to her, and handed me, a tourist in their world, the western menu. This was right in the center of Madrid. It was here, surrounded by the sensory context of her childhood, that she first opened up the story of her life to me. «The problems started when I was twelve»—Actually they had started much earlier, in her

DOI: 10.4324/9781003261490-10

family of origin, but at that time we were still getting to know each other. During those monthly meals in *her* Chinese restaurants, we were constructing without realizing it, what we would soon christen the time machine! NASA's engineers would probably have been impressed. Yao Lu traveled before my eyes, as if silent beams were opening portals to her Far Eastern memories, to her faraway childhood, and the words seemed to pour out with ease. So many memories, sometimes simply of everyday life, were stored up, wanting to come out and be shared.

On one of those days, the sight of a man next to us making angry gestures at the waitress, took our girl back to a hotel in China, during the first nights with her adoptive mother. They had both communicated in signs and motions too. Unable to speak the same language, they both turned to a primary mimicry to communicate. Her mother taught her the numbers, and through their gesticulations they began to understand each other. In school, once she got to Spain at the age of 8 or 9, she had gone through much of the same. I was sharing something of her experience, groping around in a world of meaningless utterances. A family who ate beside us seemed to be catapulted back to the faraway continent as they attentively watched a movie on the restaurant's television. A man lashed a girl's hands and back with a bamboo cane. «They hit you like that on your hand and leave you a bruise, and you can bleed», Yao Lu pointed out as if she were taking out items from her baggage to show me.

She laughed when the family seated beside us did wind up doing exactly that, as if she understood everything.

A *false self* was never far, as it was a fundamental way for her to cope with her present (and past) circumstances. I had to proceed with caution, and my daily reports to our director began to lengthen, including more and more details about my impressions and cultural travels.

It was quite the experience for me. I was in Madrid, yet I traveled with her to other worlds. This involved yielding power and certainty. I had to board the train of not-knowing, yet remain alert to enjoy a journey that opened windows to her past. It colored her present. The work in those restaurants became voyages to a faraway place that our time machine took us to instantly. Until then, Yao Lu had repudiated her origins. Thanks to the increasing Chinese immigration to Madrid, we were able to submerge ourselves in a context of tastes, scents, and sounds that could evoke some of Yao Lu's primary experiences.

We were also the object of much curiosity, and of suspicion, especially me. On more than one occasion, I felt the paternalism of the Chinese community through inquisitive and protective stares, as they looked out for the unknown girl. Who was I? What was I doing with her? They seemed to doubt the legitimacy of our meals and it made sense. «What was this teenage girl doing with an adult man who was obviously not her father? ». As calmly as I could, I took note of the menacing looks that were part of the atmosphere. And of course, although Yao Lu's skill greatly surpassed mine, we tackled our food with chopsticks! An order of pan-fried dumplings suddenly landed us in the ancient country one day, when she emphatically stated,

> This is the taste of China.

Spurred by her memories, a new curiosity was taking root. Although Yao Lu embraced the exploration of her origins, she could not find any smiles there. Still, we listened to music and what we imagined were the hits in Asia at the time; she also searched for Chinese lullabies. But as she sometimes had pointed out, perhaps our girl was now more Spanish than Chinese.

We stumbled upon references to Buddha online and read what we found to each other. She was absorbed by the resonance of her cultural history. We came across the tradition of handing over a red envelope with ideograms at the end of the year. A distant memory flickered back to life. It was supposed to bring good luck and to be given to a younger member of the family, so why not give it a shot? She wanted to get her hands on one: «I'm going to do that on Chinese New Year!».

She said it with such conviction that it seemed to be part of a core memory. I searched the stores of the Chinese community in Madrid until I found some. I purchased two; one to give her, and another so she could give it to someone as a gift herself.

The New Year was the year of the Ox, a symbol of strength and determination, so we were going to make the best of it. As I got out of my car one morning with the two recently purchased red envelopes in my hand, a young Chinese boy, absentmindedly walking to school under the weight of his book bag, noticed. He was transfixed, in a wide-eyed expression of utmost surprise, his arching eyebrows just about ready to fuse with his hairline. Such was his astonishment, that he couldn't take his eyes off the envelopes, and for an instant I feared that he might become "one" with a nearby lamppost. We were on to something culturally important!

When I handed Yao Lu her envelopes, she exclaimed loudly: «Thank you, thank you, thank you!». Together we continued our travels by going to libraries of Asian culture, where we found books, music, and a wide range of information. One day, sitting on the floor, at the foot of the library bookshelf, as the teenager she was, she flew back in time yet again: «Look Javier, the funny monkey! He's very famous!», and she explained in detail that he was a well-known cartoon character in China, as she found bits of herself through her childhood memories. We also went to a photography exhibition on Chinese women, and as I suspected, it opened a portal to her world within. She asked me to take a picture of her in front of a giant image of young fighters, like her, though these young women carried rifles in their hands. As I snapped the shot, she was pointing at them as if she were pointing at a deep and resilient part of her self.

10.1.2 Happy new year

I picked up Yao Lu early that day, so we could begin our longest trip yet to the faraway continent. As we arrived and ran up the stairs to the Palacio de los Deportes (an indoor sporting arena in Madrid also used for concerts), we could already hear the loud dance of the Dragon. With wide-eyed excitement, she wanted to take everything in; and there was a lot going on! «Look Javier! They're all Chinese!»—As two men play-acted a fight, the dragon snaked around through the crowd and acrobats appeared whilst the music reverberated. We were swallowed into the crowd, traveling into the depths of Asia. She was fascinated. She grabbed and tugged at my arm briefly; letting go to grab a red envelope that was being handed to her, then holding on again to avoid losing me, pulling on my jacket as the flow rushed us towards a stack of incomprehensible newspapers.

Had I made a mistake and made a wrong turn on the space/time highway? We were suddenly in China, that was for sure. Our girl was chuckling and told me: «It's just that they all speak in Chinese and I don't understand!» Where was the Great Wall? Yao Lu was happy, and for an instant she was mesmerized by the sight of a family with a little girl beside us. She was perhaps seven years old, about the age Yao Lu's memories went back to. Soon the musical spectacle began and Yao Lu was spellbound. She laughed on cue with everyone else. I intuited that perhaps more than anything else, it was about her wish to feel embraced, to be a part of the moment and, at least for an instant, belong. When fatigue took its toll, she asked to go back to the Home, and we set out on the trip back. As we went up the steps between the bleachers, we were surrounded by Asian faces, looking forwards doubling over in laughter and amazement. It was hard to spot a westerner. Yao Lu had never, since her adoptive trip to Madrid, been immersed among so many Chinese. Neither had I. In fact … I wondered about the construction work taken on by our mayor Gallardón! (Gallardón has been termed the Pharaoh of Madrid, after the pharaoh-like construction projects undertaken during his term in office). Was it possible that one of the bridges had been built all the way to China? But we opened the doors, and were soon walking through our familiar Madrid back to the Home, so close yet at the same time so far.

10.1.3 The experience of her experience

I spoke of how her life had changed, how much progress she had made, and we reflected together on key moments and experiences. This offered her an alternative image of herself in the context of the relationship. But more fundamentally, these could be understood as "narrative building exercises" that helped her develop a history on which to build a sense of self.[1] This would give the flexibility and the space to reflect and to construct a more authentic self as she took greater ownership of her past (Bromberg, 1996). It would stand in contrast to the dissociated, disintegrated fragments of pain and emptiness locked in an eternal present that had been scattered about her psyche. Instead of being covered over by the "mask of smiles" these fragments were now being threaded together by words that communicated (her) with others. Pointing out the achievement of these developmental milestones provided a historical thread necessary to hold her self together.

One day, a different smile, a tearful smile, accompanied her as she told me that she felt proud of herself. As she heard me describe how she had changed, she felt herself to be a person, free, happy to be a mother, and to be struggling on her path. In essence, she felt proud of being who she was. Proud! For a person crushed by abuse, whose self-esteem had withered in neglect, her statement was truly important. Yao Lu had never felt worthy of feeling and receiving affection. Her welled-up tears did not spill over that time. And they did not have to. They were now condensed in her emotions, her pride, and in her feelings of self-worth. They were the tears of change. They wrapped her in renewed strength towards the future.

Over time, with the building of our trusting relationship, she verbalized more of her wishes. The girl, who so frequently slipped away and smoothly disappeared from our conversations, was now changing. We listened to music or watched video clips together on the Home's computer as she sang along and invited me to participate. More and more, I felt myself to be a privileged guest in her inner world. *Each new day was an exhilarating trip for me.* We strolled along the paths of our shared memories. She smiled at the recollection of our past journeys during her pregnancy as she held an imaginary belly with an outstretched hand in front of her. She saw herself in the past and felt herself in the present; like someone coming out of the fog on a treacherous and winding road who, once in the clear, is liberated from having to negotiate obstacles and can sail on smoothly.

> I'm different ... I always wanted to be out on the street before. Not now.

Yao Lu was now more reflective, more thoughtful, she questioned things, including herself. She became consciously aware of the game of seduction she played with men, how she would get their attention; but it still seemed deeply anchored. She played it with me at times. But by now, it only occurred when she came back from her street escapades. Taking care to come across neither as tolerant nor as rejecting, I took care to lay out boundaries once again. At opportune moments, I pointed to the ambivalence in her messages, inviting us to pause and look at them more closely.

Yao Lu continued to grow. One afternoon she asked me if she had gone too fast with a boy she had met. I encouraged her to listen to her feelings, for her question already seemed to contain its answer. Too fast for whom? She had to find her own answer, and she was already giving herself one—«Yes».

I was able to more confidently maintain a stance of "quiet attentiveness", especially in response to crises and relapses. As she searched for herself to find her own words, instead of my own, she began to own her dilemmas, and her agency. To help her it was necessary to assist her in weaving together her present and past relations with men, without guiding her too much. I wanted to be by her side, so that she could see herself in that history, so that she could see her progress. Moreover, I had become part of that history and had as one of my goals to help clarify the differences between the language of sexual power and that of tenderness that she so often confused (see Ferenczi's concept of confusion of tongues and trauma, 1949). I had become her *resilience tutor*,[2] supporting her in her moments of success and retaining my confidence in her following her failures.

Despite the ups and downs, she gradually resumed life in the Home in more harmony. She even wanted to participate in their group activities once in a while, finding a nascent sense of belonging that had so eluded her there. She might not have been in her house, but she was in *her* Home, and she surprised me on a Spring day when, surrounded by her surrogate family, she cheerfully said:

> I've kicked out Soledad, and Hope has returned.

10.2 The disintegrating environment, fears, and flights to other worlds

On one hand, Yao Lu was more aware of her difficulties and began asking for our help; she seemed to improve quickly. On the other hand, she kept her "street self" well-defended; she avoided disclosing the locations and the identities of her abusers when she fled to the street. We were frequently frustrated at not knowing, feeling certain she was captive to unknown abusers in some dark and yet nearby corner of our city.

In time, she would return from her disappearances. Sometimes she came back escorted by agents of the national juvenile police unit (*GRUME Grupo de Menores de la Policia Nacional*, whose task was dealing with the protection of at-risk youth as well as juvenile offenders), and at other times she knocked at the door spent and exhausted. We would try to protect hope through supportive but firm boundaries. But could she make Hope truly hers? This was a frustrating period for our whole team of educators. At times I had the feeling that very few were still hopeful. Yet the most terrible thing was that at times, that small light of hope at the end of the tunnel also got blocked from view in her. It turns out that her *actings out* were no longer flights to the uncertainties of the street, but intentional visits to a decaying shanty situated between mountains of rubble, whose inhabitants sent her back to us with hellish new experiences. When we asked her where she had been, we first were wrapped in the fog of her silence. I was faced, yet again, with having to wait and exercise my patience while containing my anxiety about the uncertainties of the future.

Covered in dirt, bruised and flea-bitten, Yao Lu would return from her escapes to her broken illusions. In a Machiavellian game, her tormentor would change from a benevolent mirage she could "surrender" to into the real torturer she would have to "submit" to (Ghent, 1990).[3] She protected his identity and whereabouts from our scrutiny, and she defended him, speaking of how unfair his state of poverty was. To recognize herself as a victim to his maltreatment still proved a source of unbearable pain for her (Barudy & Dartagnan, 2005).

During this period, our girl's "mask of smiles", was not only less frequent but was also less effective in hiding her emotions. The pain that drove her acting out could no longer be dissociated. It could certainly not be ignored. Neither a «laissez-faire» attitude nor a simplistic "accepting" attitude after her acting-out were even conceivable, given the real risk of death she ran. It also made little sense to focus on setting up daily routines as a way of helping her if every time (and it was frequent) she became overwhelmed by anxiety she fled, letting herself plummet into the abyss.

Yao Lu needed limits, coherent limits that pointed out the responsibility *she* had. In dumping her breakdowns on others, in this case on me, she avoided gaining ownership of her own existence. By continuing to fling herself at her tormentors on the street, while knowing she would always be taken back in by me, by the Home, she was consolidating the cyclical and habitual dynamic of her life. She had to claim her agency however painful that may be. *Her life was hers*; that was clear enough, *but better to live it than spend it dying*. She was also getting older and my accompaniment was limited. Extending it indefinitely could have negative results, running the risk of forging a symbiotic dependence and disempowerment, contrary to the goal of our work, which was precisely for her to achieve autonomy and of a healthy independence.

After discussing the situation with our director, I went to the Home and up to her room, after Yao Lu returned from a new crisis and a new destructive flight to the shanty. I greeted her and let her know that I was glad to see she was alright, but that I was leaving, because it was she who had to think. That was now *her job*, not mine. She had to think through everything she had managed to accomplish over the past months, and it was her responsibility to consider if she could allow herself to do things differently, or if she would rather be blown about by the four winds. I was straightforward, even blunt, pointing to a dynamic over which she had to gain perspective and begin to take responsibility. Her life depended on it. After 15 minutes, I said goodbye to a girl who looked at me with a sad sigh. It was hard work. The point was not to be harsh, nor to be right, nor to break her down, but not doing something different would have been more of the same and Yao Lu needed to think. This intervention was aimed at cutting through her cyclical dynamic, and to affirm her value. The limit struck home.

The next time I saw her, I sat down calmly with a concise «Hello» letting a long and poignant silence resonate, inviting her to take responsibility for the exchanges. Several minutes followed during which she stared at me, then at the door, and then at the wall. I tapped her on the shoulder without saying a word. She immediately asked me if I was leaving, as if the long-anticipated prophecy of abandonment was confirmed. I answered with another question, giving her back the responsibility in the exchange. «Do you want me to leave?». «No». We resumed a silent non-verbal echo.

It was risky. My silence could be experienced as an act of aggression by our girl, for whom this kind of interpretation of the situation would fit her passive-aggressive coping mechanisms well. I thought she may have been going down that road, so I grabbed pen and paper, slid across the room noisily on a chair with wheels, and wrote a message in big letters. She looked at me curiously—when I looked over, she rapidly turned away—and I placed the paper on the wall where her gaze was riveted. «HELLO». She smiled, I waited ... and again silence. After a while I wrote another note. «Are you bored?» «NO», and again she smiled. I confronted her sulky silence, with my attempts at humor that were also insistent invitations for her to assume her responsibility in the dialogue.

If this went on much longer, it might turn into a fun game but it would also be repeating an old pattern. I could only point out the path, but she had to take it. I made up my mind to write one last note. «I'm going to get a drink of water and meanwhile you think about what we should talk about.» «Ok». It was directive, yet non-specific. I would do nothing more. When I got back she was ready to bravely put words to her unsteady emotions. She was wrapped in the warmth of a blanket for protective cover.

> I'm a mess. My life sucks.

She was choking and sobbing as she spoke. She wanted for all of us to leave her alone, to abandon her so she could abandon herself to the street. The message was hard to comprehend, to say the least. How can one be sad because others do not allow them to jump into the abyss? I responded by articulating the contradictory messages between her facial expression and her words, thus clarifying the fear that was driving her desire to flee.

She spoke in tears of her maltreatment. She spoke of China, of how she felt that I had been angry with her the previous day, and of being sad. Affectionately, I reflected aloud on the importance for her to take responsibility for what she could only do herself. My message had hit home. But she continued to fight off and struggle against the will to become the agent of her life. Turmoil, smiles, tears, punctuated the giant steps forwards and the setbacks. For Yao Lu, in Dickens's phrase, «It was the best of times, it was the worst of times, it was the age of wisdom, it was the age of foolishness, it was the epoch of belief, it was the epoch of incredulity, it was the season of Light, it was the season of Darkness, it was the Spring of hope, it was the Winter of despair, we had everything before us, we had nothing before us» (Dickens, 1921).

In just a few words, she managed to sum up her tormented existence:

> I like being abused, but not all the time.

It was the period of antitheses: of sun and rain, of smiles and tears, of confusion and increasing clarity, of reflection and blind enactments. Her return to the shanty still seemed to be something inevitable, but the opposing sides of the turmoil were being experienced closer together, perhaps one day to be more fully integrated was the hope.

10.2.1 Connecting with the lost child

After returning from one of my breaks, we resumed the work from the last time she ran away. A couple of days before I left, she had disappeared. Perhaps she wanted me to know that if I was not going to be there, neither would she.

We went for a walk in a nearby park and sat by a playground. I was tactful in my inquiry. And I asked about her secret. Without my making much of an effort, she began to talk more openly, as if a very protected part of herself were struggling to come out into the light of day. She picked up a stick and she began to draw geometrical figures in the sand. The result was a map. She shared memories as she drew. I observed her elegant movements, looking on in curiosity and patiently asking her to explain the details that lay before me, and I kept a mental picture, just in case. She was telling me where her infamous shanty that she ran away to was. Though still protective of that world, she was revealing, however indirectly, the unknown whereabouts she ran to. It was as if some small and resilient part of herself were reaching out to me to take care of her when in crisis.

This brave inner part had made appearances in the past, for instance during her relations with Marcelo. In her dreams, she appeared as a fighting ninja, vehemently battling against evildoers with a sword. She spoke of the swordsman as if it was a part of her, and yet not; both distant and close.

During the weeks prior to the drawing of the map, I had been scouting out diverse neighborhoods where I thought the "shanty" might be. I knew Yao Lu frequented the world of marginal juveniles in the neighborhoods of North African immigrants, so I went into Arabic-accented cafeterias, where I understood little and was welcomed by suspicious stares. I had to be very careful about asking about her, because I could put her in danger. I had to be careful for both our sakes. I was hesitant about disclosing the reason for my inquiries; I feared that could trigger a beating if I did not find her first. I sensed I was very close, because her prior descriptions fit the area I was in.

I knocked on the doors of houses in ruins and walked down alleyways and passed dark corners without success; managing as best I could under the heavy artillery of deadly stares and suspicious murmurs. I was repeatedly offered hashish. I was seen as a consumer, or even a policeman. As I renewed my searches for our girl, I gradually became a habitual figure. I was confident I knew how to move around in dicey places, but nevertheless doing so was a risk. I arrived at a small plaza, amidst furtive glances and quickened paces. There was an Internet call center at the rear of the place, I went in to ask and ... bingo! The owners knew her. They seemed relieved to be able to pour out their concern to me, for they saw her frequently. Sometimes she went into their call center, other times she would sit on a bench in front of the window, surrounded by a group of young men and adolescents who mocked and laughed at her. They denigrated her through displays of sexualized contempt. The owners told me that she responded by lowering her head under the onslaught.

I felt like a cartographer of her experiential map, and now she had bravely taken the lead. She had drawn it out in the sand to show me her hideout. On the day of a new disappearance, I got a call from the Home; Yao Lu had been on her way back from her mother's house, but had spent the night out and was nowhere to be found. They were concerned, as was I. I set off to find her.

Amidst the back and forth of her crises and improvements, our girl had started to see a friendly guy with whom she had connected over the Internet. She had already introduced me to him. In fact, she had wanted to do so when he came to pick her up one day, and I stayed overtime so we could meet. He seemed nice enough. We had spoken about him a great deal, and I had witnessed how she instant messaged with him on various occasions. Yao Lu urgently sought advice from me. «What do I say? What do I do?». And I would respond: «What do you feel?».

That weekend she had received permission to go out with some "girl friends" but had gone out with this boy instead. She came back to the Home by the curfew, smiling and happy at the success of her little ploy. This kind of normal defiance of authority was almost welcome, though we would have preferred for her to direct a bit more of it towards her tormentors rather than her caregivers. The following day she went to her mother's house and, hoping perhaps to connect and to be understood, maybe also as a way of ridding herself from the guilt of tricking us, she let her mother know. But instead of supporting Yao Lu for opening up to her, she reprimanded her, and immediately they were both in the grips of the old fears, mistrust, and apprehensions. Amidst rage and tears, all the improvements were swept away as if by a tsunami. And the mother's premonition that nothing would ever change turned into a self-fulfilling reality. It confirmed her prophecy about our girl's inability to be taken care of, to be mothered, and they were both thrown back into a dynamic of mutual powerlessness, failure, and resentment. Instead of going back to the Home on her own, Yao Lu went straight down the path of pseudosecurity and pain to the shanty, where she could find the misery of her origins. It was in these (emotional) places that her submissive identity had been forged, and where sex offered her a (false) refuge.

I was getting ready to go out in search of her again. I tried to be calm. I took my time, turned on the computer, and reread my notes about the map drawn in the sand. I opened up Google maps as I had a general idea of what I was looking for. With enough patience, I came across what seemed a likely spot, the remains of some old dwellings, shanties, between the trees and debris of what seemed like a vacant lot. I got into my car and there I went.

10.2.2 Visits to the underworld and the games of power

I sailed through the traffic riding the wave of anxiety, trying to be as aware of my fears as possible, trying to maintain perspective and to not be paralyzed by them. I do not remember what music came over the radio. Sometimes when I searched for her I listened to rap with a driving bass and an empowering message to give me strength, but internally, I was frenetic.

I felt vulnerable out in the open in unfamiliar territory, not knowing what I was going to find. This precarious world into which our troubled girl disappeared, and which spit her back out trembling and bruised, could be dangerous. I parked at a safe distance in the general neighborhood and began to wade deep into my fears, amidst the barren hills and lifeless rubble. Attempting to remain calm, I deliberately walked along dirt paths that wove into one another, through fields of discarded washing machines and garbage. My heart was going faster than my feet. Calm down! I recalled the map and, putting it together with her descriptions, I arrived in front of an old run-down abandoned-looking house. There were actually cars parked behind a large green gate and I peeked in, but I couldn't see anyone. I would come back and ring the bell, but first it was best to scout out the area, lest I find myself in need of a quick exit. I continued down the dirt path a few steps and saw the remnants of the wall of an old hut rise before me. They looked like ruins jutting out over a mountain of rubble. Surely, nobody could live there; the conditions were miserable. A spring breeze was blowing, and I realized that a worn-out sheet, strung out over the remnants of the wall, was flapping in the wind. It was less than two meters away, but it had seemed to me just another scrap of the chaotic mountain of debris. My eyes, unaccustomed to see amidst the arsenal of refuse, were over-stimulated by the sheer amount of disorderly objects. And my heartbeat was in the grips of a fast-paced jazz. I took a better look and discovered a long cable, stretched out to the neighboring shanty; an unmistakable sign of life in the ruins!

To get a better look, I peered in over the pile of cement, old bricks, legless dolls, broken toys, mixed with empty bottles and cans. A dog started to bark and seconds later a North African looking man of about 35 came out from the filth, barefoot and bare-chested. He seemed an extremely strong individual, although I would later realize that the impression was the product of the rush of anxiety more than anything else. I realized that I was encountering my fears, mine and no one else's, and that allowed me to regain some control and work amidst them.

I greeted him with a show of confidence from my position on the pile of rubble, which allowed me an excellent view of that *kingdom*: a lot full of fish heads, empty *liter bottles* of liquor, and various remnants of empty and broken containers.

—Hello I'm Javier, do you know an Asian girl named Yao Lu?
—Yes, she's inside, come in.
—No, no, thank you! Better you tell her to come out please, that I'm here to visit her.
—Yao Luúú, Jaaaavier is here looking for you!... Yao Luúú!

That was the start. I could see we had initiated a power game, on his turf. And it could get tricky. I decided to get down from my vantage point, having to negotiate the brush, the thorny bushes, and low-lying trees that hugged the wall, but remaining cautious, as he again invited me in. The environment was clearly dangerous; I had to manage but still listen to my fear.

I stepped over the carpet of cans and bottles that gave a new texture to the mud that had absorbed them. In four strides, I found myself facing a lost world, once only a temporary map in the sand. Decisively, I held out my hand to that guy, not without the urge to crush it paper-thin. I automatically asked how he was doing, and noted a hint of fearful surprise that he struggled to disguise. That was a potential advantage. I had to play my hand carefully, recognize my own fears, and have them pass undetected while still listening to them for my own protection. It was obvious I was not expected, and this too was part of my advantage. He asked me if I was «from the facility», and quickly a torrent of words and explanations came pouring out of him. He assured me he took good care of Yao Lu, notwithstanding that sometimes she appeared and remained with him for a day, two or three days on occasion, or he might not see her for a month until, once again, she reappeared, so he was there for her, and so on and so forth.

I was aware of *what his care entailed.* All these urgent explanations and verbose answers to unasked questions echoed in my racing mind.

More than the contents, it all spoke to how tense the situation was, and that it was important to diffuse it and leave as soon as possible.

He picked up some panties tossed at the edge of the pile of rubble and tried to hand them to me, stating they were clean. «NO! Give them back to Yao Lu». It was a disgusting invitation to join him in some way in the invasion of our girl. Boundaries were absent here. I walked with him through the misery that flanked the path to his house, to the precarious threshold of the fortress of our girl's fears. If *Soledad* were to live somewhere, it was here. I am sure. Too bad she was invisible! There was no door to the shack, more like a tall construction fence, with an old rug hanging over it. He invited me in, but I was alone, and I did not do so. I had to stay constantly alert, monitoring and controlling myself while monitoring him with a vigilant eye, in the dangerous dance of mistrust unfolding between us.

In unstable and risky situations like this one, my own façade of security could be interpreted as a show of dominance and could subtly destabilize the other. I had experienced it before. It had to be a subtle exercise, on one hand not backing down in fear, but also allowing for the other to retain a certain sense of control. If he felt threatened and if his fears were exposed, he could launch some kind of attack. I had to find the balance between dominance and submission. Losing it would be a disaster. I had to speak from a centered and confident place. Having been able to process my own fears, hopefully, I had to attempt to destabilize my enemy «just a little», without overdoing it, keeping him just a bit off balance and on his heels to avoid an aggressive/defensive reaction. I could also not let him see my fear. If he perceived me to be intimidated and powerless in the relationship, although it would not destabilize him, it could also invite violence. On the other hand, to walk on that tightrope involved giving back to him at least some illusion of control, like an acrobat using gravity in a smooth show of balance, each time rectifying the pull to the right, to the left, as well forward and backward. I had to stay on top of what was mine, and his as well, so we could both move about in the dance of our unstable fears, and keep our balance, so I could take Yao Lu back with me. Multiple elements to keep in mind, in a system where stability was extremely fragile, like free-form jazz! It was no small feat, and the demands for self-control were exacting, as I worked to slow down the *tempo*.

Our girl appeared from out of the deepest darkness, and I was glad I had decided not to go in. Respecting her privacy was important, even in the lugubrious corners of that underworld. When he opened the fence a little wider to let her out, I saw a little girl peer out as if landing from another galaxy, one of threadbare mattresses without sheets, thrown on the ground, a feeding ground for rats. He handed over her underwear and I looked away, stepping aside a little too, allowing for privacy in a world without it.

His fears began to spike: «Are you taking her to the facility? Are you going to the facility?». Prudently, I just stalled not really answering him, while moving our girl along that black hole through to the present. I let her know I was glad to see her, that I had worried about her. In calm silence, we retraced the paths through the empty lot together, until we got to the car. We soon reached the open doors to the Home, where they were getting ready for one of their weekly group therapy meetings with the children.

We would continue. But it was now time for me to go back to my own house and to try to put my bubbling inner world back in order. Our girl was safe. The rest of the team would take on the functions of a foster family. It was my turn to rest now, although I doubted I would be able to do so. I got to the door of my apartment, which I shared with two of my best friends and the girlfriend of one of them who was frequently there too. I entered, «Hello family!». Oh how great those words sounded!—Our routine daily greeting. They were cooking and it was now my time to try to relax, to come down from the intensity of the day. After a shared dinner, we ended up sitting in the living room to bid the day farewell. Someone had bought a new fish, a colorful new inhabitant that was getting to know his aquarium, and our home.[4]

10.2.3 Affect therapy

The next day, Yao Lu was afraid that I would be disappointed in her. She worried about what I thought of her. What did I think after seeing her in that part of the underworld? How would that change our relationship? The question was a good one that I had already asked myself over long hours. She must have gone through a very rough time to go back to a place like that, and I invited her to remember my first words that day: «I'm glad to see you, are you ok?». They touched her and Yao Lu's eyes welled-up. «It's just that since you played dumb and like you didn't know, when I told you where the shanty was», she said in reference to the day of her drawings in the sand. To emotionally contain her while remaining aware of all that was going on was clearly impossible for me.

She said she had doubted that I would go look for her, and she also said she was sure that I would. That was why she drew for me that day, in the sand in the playground. In fact, she thanked me for going, for she felt trapped and bewildered there, unable to leave.

Affectionately, I wrapped my arm around her shoulders as I said: «You're welcome, Yao Lu». She smiled, saying she felt embarrassed. By my going to search for her all the way in the darkest corners of lost worlds, I hoped that a sense of her own self-worth got through. The firmly held belief that she was not fit to be loved, not fit for affection, might weaken, eventually to be disproved.

She spoke a great deal that afternoon. She told me how she felt pangs of pain when her mother said something negative, how her already low self-esteem sank even lower whenever her mother distrusted her, and how she felt undeserving of a better life, despite seeing the possibilities before her. She never received the simple, powerful, and soothing maternal message «It's going to be ok». Needless to say, she participated in fueling the feedback loop of anxiety, although little by little it seemed to be losing some steam. I want to be clear. Notwithstanding her relapses, despite the appearances, Yao Lu was improving a great deal, as well as her mother, and so was their relationship. With greater frequency, they enjoyed new moments of shared feeling and tranquility.

We spent months talking about her courageous efforts to face her fears, about how the work of her heart and mind were necessary to mitigate those fears. I often encouraged her to take off her glasses, and hand them over so I could study them in detail. I would look at them closely, then through them in both directions, onto the world and onto her world, then return them shaking my head, deducing that since she had switched to «grown up» frames, her positive changes were obviously due to that. She would burst into laughter, «That's not true!». She spoke of feeling progressively more understood by the educators, more open to the world, and to her own inner world.

In general, Yao Lu was getting to know herself more and more, as we tried to support her with basic trust, to give her the opportunity for growth, notwithstanding all of her setbacks. Some days she said she felt «peaceful» or «happy» when I asked her how she felt. She was even able to worry about me. It was a subtle and significant indication of the attachment that developed over time. It was a cool afternoon and, as we spoke about the cold, she offered me her sweater. I smiled and thanked her, kindly declining it. I was wearing my own and a slim sweater with a female cut was not my style. I was also much bigger than her! Still, it was a nice gesture, and she later reminded me that I should not catch a cold, as if I had suddenly become a child to take care of. Perhaps this was a way she had of telling me that she appreciated our conversations and that I was not allowed to miss them, though she had told me that more explicitly before.

Months later, in the midst of the light September rains, I reminded her to wear a raincoat on our walk, and she told me: «I don't care if I get wet». «Yes, Yao Lu, but I do care if you get wet». With a slight and affectionate smile, she said: «Some days I take care of you and others you take care of me», and off she went to her room to get a coat for our outing, though the important blanket was one of care.

10.2.4 Navigating through rough emotional seas

Perhaps the most difficult thing for me during this turbulent period was handling my own emotions. I had to be conscious of them and ensure that they did not derail our relationship of accompaniment. As much as possible, they should be put to therapeutic use. I could not «cease to react» before her, but the fact that I was aware of them increased the chances that I could do so more adequately.[5] Following her repeated flights to that horrible dwelling, I was overcome by fury, impotence, and despair. I wanted to run from my anxiety, turn it into anger. What a difficult task it was, to work on oneself by oneself! But, how necessary and important all the same! Many a time, I felt pulled into her anxiety, drawn to let myself be taken over by the to and fro of her temperament, but I had to keep my balance. I strove to think before I spoke, to give myself time and space. I worked to ensure that I was responding, not just reacting emotionally, and staying aware of my own emotions. I felt all the anxiety she provoked in me. My insides churned.

I shared the whole burden with my director, who helped me put it into context and understand it. She provided suggestions and clarified nuances. She invited me to think and to accept my feelings. She guided me through so many experiences from a place of calm and hopeful critique; so that I not feel rushed, and that I patiently respect Yao Lu's pace. I always felt her to be present with constant and firm support in our weekly emails and meetings. She did the same with the rest of the professionals on our team.

I felt urges to act, to respond, or simply to run away from these emotions closing in on me, to turn away, when *what I had to do was to be present and to listen.* I worked through my *countertransference.* Our relationship had to survive these torments, my torments, although they were also an echo of hers. I had *to be a safe haven in her chaos,* and in spite of her *transferences,* I had to be tolerant and to take care of her. I thought things over, silently and mindfully, hanging on to the echoes of emotions that were mine, and the work continued.

I had recently read an article on childhood sexual abuse and the therapist's experience in a specific case (Abad, 2001). I identified with many of the therapist's intense experiences. My accompaniment was tough going and when the emotional atmosphere was one of abuse, it frequently sent me home stirred up and feeling ill, where I needed to settle down and get reorganized. Some days, angry and wailing, she attacked, stating that she no longer wanted to see me again, that I should leave. She generally did this when the end of our session had come, or when I sensed it was best to shorten it that day. She would then try to turn me into a bad guy who hurt her. I always replied that I would be there as usual on the following day, to continue our work. Affectionately, I would lay my hand on her head before I left.

She ran away many times, and as I described earlier when I took a leave of absence, it was as if she were trying to let me know how painful it was, and how abandoned she felt.

I often found myself worrying about her, mulling over problems we had been working on or thinking about the steps we had taken throughout her process. At the same time, theories, authors, instructors, resonated in the distance of lecture rooms, and I had a hard time paying attention to them. It seemed that her identity could do nothing but crumble on its weight, since it was so diluted in the other person. Our relationship could not sustain her all the time. Nevertheless, I remained available, and she had my number. But it was not enough. Be it as it may, on certain occasions she would reappear upon my return, and our work would continue slowly forging a secure base from which to explore her self and assume the emotional risks yet again (Bowlby, 1988).

On other days she would attack me with cutting aggression, flinging at me that although I knew a lot about what had happened in her life, I knew nothing of her suffering or what she felt. I stayed there, sharing and tolerating her pain, by way of support and holding. I was frequently invaded by a deep resentment at the injustice she had faced. Worry and frustration that our time was running out also visited me occasionally. This frustration did not take over my relationship with her, but I did feel her anxiety and somehow made it my own, constantly re-digesting it in my work with her. I did not throw it back at her. It was too much.

I found myself going out for longer runs each day during my free afternoons, or searching for a gym that would allow me to burn off the tension to keep it under control. Saying goodbye frightened me. Was I so different from our girl then? At that time, I was attending a Balint[6] group, which was available for training and emotional support of the therapeutic educators of our team, and it also allowed me to reduce some of the tensions I carried on my burdened shoulders. But since some colleagues already knew Yao Lu, I felt protective and I was restricted in what I could say. Supervision was effective and helpful, though a personal therapy would have been even more useful, but at that point, just like for many others, it scared me! It was difficult to admit, so I "took" care of myself» as best I knew how, between exercise, the individual and group supervisions in the context of work, and dinners with my "family".

Staying calm in the midst of her emotional chaos was important, and it was impossible to do so without first being at peace myself. Although I pushed her at times, I always tried to be respectful of her pace, advancing slowly in my inquiry and in my expectations. I felt sadness at a world I wished to be very different. *In our day-to-day work to bolster our girl's resiliencies, I also grew increasingly aware of my own.* I saw my difficulties but also began to discern my strengths, growing and maturing just as she did. Her increasing capacity to verbalize and share her experience was important to her maturing. And she was.

> I want to talk with girls that have been through the same things
> I have and that they be my best friends.

But sometimes Soledad returned and our girl felt anxious, exuding despair once again. «I want to wipe myself off the map», she said one day as she looked up at a big map hanging on the wall beside her. I told her: «Don't bother searching, you won't spot yourself there. And you won't find me either», and she answered in a loud «Javieeer!», as we both broke into laughter, crossing a bridge of resilience.

A more dramatic moment took place after one of her returns, when I found her lying on the bed in her room, flooded by deep despair. She opened her eyes and in a serious, yet animated tone, I told her: «Hello Yao Lu. I know you've been out, and that you came back with the police. Do you want to talk about your problems or not? You decide». «Yes». «Then let's go. I'll only wait for you for five minutes, sitting outside». Yao Lu did come out, but did not go to sit in her chair, situated in front of mine. She went into the adjacent bathroom. The act could seem like a minor event, but that day, she left the door cracked open.

I was seated, which allowed her enough privacy because the door was not right in front of me and was only slightly open. But I felt abruptly flooded by a surge of rage. I was furious. She dumped the recent behaviors of abuse she had submitted herself to, all over me. Visceral anger emerged in me, and I felt the pressure to act accordingly and assert my dominance in some way—to explode, to be harsh, like a man, as had so many men in Yao Lu's life. Though I felt provoked, I was able to tolerate it without acting out, but I admit that my first impulse was to get up and close the bathroom door, maybe slam it shut. I was now more aware of this, just as I was of our girl's need to feel that I could tolerate my own feelings and not react impulsively in the role of abuser she was trying to induce in me during those moments.

I thus allowed myself to slide back into a therapeutic stance, a sort of "therapeutic surrender" (Ghent, 1990) in which my subjectivity could become part of a transitional space (Winnicott, 1971) for the metabolizing and reabsorbing of what was intolerable for Yao Lu

(Bion, 1990), and gradually we could co-construct a different relationship marked by thirdness (Benjamin, 2004), where we could truly "meet" one another. I could then see that it was perhaps her way of having me feel the invasion and abuse she had just recently felt. Life in the shanty was like that, invasive, rushed, with no privacy. I had seen it myself! It was hard![7]

It was a challenge, maybe set up to see how I would handle my anxiety. I did not act out and take it out on her. I "sat with it" and contained it. A few minutes later, she sat before me. I kept silent. Yao Lu needed to play out her experience of abuse, and she needed me to tolerate it, so hopefully she might be able to tolerate her own experience, and eventually work through it. It took an enormous effort for her to start, but she willingly remained sitting in front of me. My silence could have meant many things to her, but by remaining present and containing my anxiety, I intended to convey that I was here to listen because she wanted to talk, and that here was her space to do so.

She looked at me incredulously, as if she could not believe that I did not react. I did not know, but I remained silent. I got up unhurriedly, slowly opened the blinds a little more, and sat back down. Perhaps it was simply a situation where the complementarity of how we each dealt with anxiety got played out in the relationship, in which she projected and I endured. At that point, I really just didn't quite know what else I could say or do. So I "gave up" my anger and "surrendered" to the encounter, not knowing what it all would bring. I felt, she felt, I lived, she lived, and in the interaction and intermingling of our emotions, but of separate subjectivities, we were able to find together a new place of calm for us both. We both survived, but we survived together! Benjamin (2004) referred to this as the «moral third», or «third in the one». After a settling silence, she said «It's just that I don't know what it is you want me to say. That I could care less about everything?».

We could talk about that if she wanted, but she had to decide for herself. Little by little, doors began to open, and she spoke about not caring about anything; that she did not care if she turned 18 or 20.

> Would you like to stay seventeen?
>   Yes!

The fears of becoming an adult had arrived. She explained that, if she froze at seventeen, there would always be people around her, people to help her. We were connecting to a key fear, one which spoke directly to how her fear of abandonment prevented her from assuming responsibility for her life.

She had come out from her room to talk, so I invited her to be brave. I could see her eyes teeming with tears as she began to speak of the abandonment she felt when she talked with her mother who, tired of her behavior, had refused to come to see her today. She said she felt emotionally volatile, swinging from highs to lows. We spoke of rules of self-care, and principles of self-regulation, of not having had them, nor even wanting them, and preferring to fling herself at the extremes with abandon.

But even in her hurricanes, Yao Lu wanted to preserve some of the comforts of moderation. She liked hot showers, and clean clothes, perhaps tossed around the floor, but clean nonetheless, so she wouldn't step on them! Rule number one: Humor![8] It was humor that helped us both to keep hope in front of the incommensurable tensions between her wishes and the reality of her life. Humor helped us "transform that hidden pain, in digested pain and integrate it into the fabric of her life" (Vanistendael, 2004, p.125 author's translation). We frequently used humor. Here we likened her room to an orchard, where she would walk around and pick clothes to wear from ground-hugging bushes and low-lying vines, if it was allowed. She would be forced to walk about her room in a sort of tribal dance without music to avoid stepping on anything of value.

She had begun to shake herself free from her shackles and she expressed realistic wishes to have a stable job someday, even an apartment of her own. It reflected normal aspirations of a girl her age. I contrasted them lightheartedly to the shanty world. «I want a big apartment! And a big desk!». I quickly added: «And I'm sure a large stuffed animal!». «Yes!». «Like in the shanty?», and she laughed wholeheartedly, as the residual tensions melted with the humor. I suggested that maybe the shanty's rats, in spite of being large and furry, were not good friends or comfortable cuddly toys. «Noooo!!». The laughter became a fit of laughter. The humor helped replace tearful sadness and horror with a resilient hope for a better life.

We knew that the fears of coming of age (18) were here. They can be especially acute, even debilitating for abandoned children, who feel they come from nowhere and have nowhere to go. The feeling of not belonging dogged Yao Lu everywhere she went, and her despair turned into self-destructive impulses that wreaked havoc.

Our director and I had already spoken of this looming date, and we decided that the time had come to tell Yao Lu that the doors of our therapeutic center would remain open after the (*feared* and longed for) 18th birthday if she so wished. She was asked to think it over and I believe she let out a great inward sigh in hearing our proposal. It was not evident, but it seemed that her anxiety dissipated. For a moment at least, the whirling maelstrom abated and she found a place where she could belong. She remained thoughtful, traveling about her inner world. «See you next time Javier ...», and I left.

10.2.5 Lost messages

What was established is what I call an emotional dynamic equilibrium. Far from being a fixed state, the equilibrium is *dynamic*, with fluctuating emotions and moods. These, however, are contained within less dramatic and chaotic limits, hence a (relative) equilibrium, which allows for exploration and reflection. The peaks and the valleys were more moderate, less dangerous, and thus became amenable to understanding, and acceptance, as part of her growth process. During one of those days when Yao Lu was sad and blue, we took the opportunity to revisit her wish to relive her childhood, a wish that ran through the story of her life. Within the bounds of this dynamic equilibrium, the emotions could be used as a springboard for productive exploration, as opposed to a crisis when the goal became to simply regulate them. Yao Lu viewed herself as a sad and long-suffering girl, in permanent search of a (fantasized) lost state of happiness. This happiness could be found in unintegrated fragments she had felt momentarily at times in the past, so I asked about her positive experiences in her recollections of China. We constructed a setting in which to invite child Yao Lu into the present with the help of memories that brought her to life. Shortly thereafter, on a vibrant pink chair, the memory of petite Yao Lu of the past sat right there by our side. What might she have in store for us?

We brought that little girl back to life in our conversation, a little girl forgotten for long periods, yet still very much alive. She was a resilient fighter, and with great capacity for growth. We invited her to join our conversation, cradling little Yao Lu in her memory through to the soothing present. It was nice to feel how we were reaching original parts of herself, parts that had to do with Yao Lu's foundational resiliencies in the face of continued, hard, and profound injustices in her life. I accompanied her in this journey, drawing memories from the past into the present to make her strong. The image in her mind was of eight-year-old Yao Lu, and we gradually gave her form so she could sit in the pink chair in front of us. Yao Lu spoke of a time of emotional support, of love, of the affection of a foster family back there in her remote China. We traveled to the past as we spoke, anchored in the present of that afternoon in Madrid.

What was this eight-year-old Yao Lu like?

Capricious...

What do you mean by capricious?

That she wanted lots of things.

What things? Any in particular she liked very much? Stuffed animals...?

Yes. A duck.

And what was that duck like?

It had feathers, yellow, and an orange beak... And you pressed it, and it said quack-quack. [Yao Lu was smiling, though with nostalgic sadness].

And what else was that girl like?

Intelligent.

Intelligent. That girl was intelligent was she?

Yes. And studious, she liked books a lot... [Yao Lu started to describe how her mother helped her study. She spoke of a Yao Lu as a fighter who doesn't quit.]

And what did that little Yao Lu in China need?

A large family. Affection... love...

A large family, with lots of brothers and sisters, so she could get lots of affection from all around?

Yes.

As we brought the Yao Lu of China to life, she was able to express her unmet emotional needs, and assert her strengths. We invited her to come visit us, so both Yao Lus could sit across each other. No longer recalled from memory, this little girl from China took her own powerful space, propelling Yao Lu forward in this present future of hers. The advice was in the voice of a teenager, but it resonated with the deep wisdom of her lived past.

And would you have anything to suggest to this little girl so she can keep it in mind? [It was interesting, because when I said this, Yao Lu stretched out her foot and began gently caressing the chair]

That she...

Remember, tell her, she's sitting over there.

That you listen ... that you don't do anything nuts ... [She said it a few more times, the last one with more force and intensity ...]

Can you think of anything else you would like to tell her?

YOU SHOULD FIGHT!!!

[She smiled earnestly, as she was getting her message through to a resilient and hidden part within herself]

She recognized herself in the needs and challenges of that little girl, and they awoke together through the words of encouragement, strength, and invitations to persevere. Yao Lu was lighting up from strengths coming from her inner recesses: «You should fight!». A simple and powerful message, about her, for her: You should fight, Yao Lu!

10.2.6 Tears of joy and the experience of growth

We were building on the shoulders of Hope (Esperanza), but it was not always easy to find her... «Should we text her? Does she have a cellphone?». Our girl would abandon herself to laughter, and we returned to a world where improvement was possible. We laughed a lot, even when the times were tough.

Somehow, amidst the flickers of humor, we reconnected with the hopeful world of infancy, and with its magic, both of us recharged with strengths. "You see (reader) when the first baby laughed for the first time, its laugh broke into a thousand pieces, and they all went skipping about, and that was the beginning of fairies." (James Mathew Barrie, 1911, Ch. 3). And it was precisely with that world that we tried to connect, full of dreams and flickering Hopes, where success was made possible, and where Yao Lu might come out from her torments.

It has always been my belief that, when abandoning oneself to the contractions of humor, the little forgotten child in us emerges through the years and layers of an adult face, greeting us from within, in a «Yes, I am here. And I am still alive!». It's as if one can see a light in the wholehearted laughter of friends, the light of Hope (Esperanza). When laughter is genuine, people shine. If one has the good fortune of keeping friends from childhood, laughter returns old playmates to each other, unchanged by the inexorable passage of time.

We were both sailing, with passports and visas, between two worlds, past and present, in quest of the future. I encouraged our girl to dramatize and act out her experience, including unsteadiness of a baby attempting to get up and stand. She tottered and fell back down again. I participated by inviting her with an outstretched hand to get up from the chair. She mimicked a wobbling baby, falling into her seat and trying it again. She laughed, smiled, and laughed again, stating that this is how she felt then. We would support her back then. We believed in her and we would encourage her in taking her first steps again. But towards where? What did she want to resolve? «The thing about running away and being in the street». As she told me sobbing one day, her problem was essentially in her relationship with men, a sly game she still felt unable to keep under control, an unconscious game that propelled her headlong into her life-long nightmare, to "wake up" bruised, used and sad.

What I could do as just her educator and therapeutic companion was woefully limited. I was not a magician, but maybe she could take something with her from the Home, from us. The twilight of her stay with us was nearing. Time kept passing inexorably by, and she could not remain indefinitely. As we walked under the trees of a park, I asked her about what she might want to take away: «The affection, being in charge of my life». But, how could those intangible yet so heartfelt gifts be wrapped up? «Here, inside», and she pointed at her chest, framing it in a beautiful and deep smile.

We gifted her an unselfish bond for the calm and ongoing reconstruction of her life; an attachment that would not react aggressively when faced with her temperamental outbursts; a bond that would not bind her to the old injuries she repeatedly tried to escape, that would allow her to gradually rescript the story of her life; to find herself in a safer and more secure environment. *That was our greatest gift.* We could wrap her up in a healthy relationship, in which she could be nurtured, in which she could heal herself in her *being* and her *becoming.* She would take responsibility, autonomy, and freedom with her! Above all she would take care, as a constant reminder of the possibility of feeling it from others and thus, from within herself. How interesting, that was the first gift she mentioned.

The flickers of happiness were more frequent during that time, and they also provided me with the necessary strength, to continue down the fraught and treacherous road between lonesome Soledad and hopeful Esperanza. Sometimes she greeted me with an ecstatic «I can do it Javier! I'm happy!», or other such envigorating statements. It is true that they sometimes seemed more like hypomanic jumps of joy than genuine happiness, but our girl had to learn how to temper herself down too. Some of the difficulties with her mother also seemed to be clearing up. The communication between them was becoming clearer and more direct. Neither of them wanted to fail in their relationship. They began to fight more as a team! More constructively.

Our girl would miss us—as we would miss her too. Worried by the possibility of never seeing us again, she told me one day, part statement, part question, fearful: «Will we be able to see each other sometime?». Sure we could!

I have to sort out my life, because sometimes I feel scared. Aaaahhh!

The thing is, freedom was scary, really scary, especially for a girl who was peering out onto new horizons from an old and wretched background of submission to the malignant and destructive abuse of others.

Her wish to be able to live autonomously, to cook, to wash her clothes, to work, and to study, all had our encouragement and support. She had always had them, but now even more so with her asking for them. She invited me for a home-cooked spaghetti meal one day, and I agreed to stay. I helped her in the kitchen, chopping up ingredients, allowing her to diligently give me direction like a high-class chef. The meal was excellent! I had seconds!

It was also important to highlight the impact of her changes, her own power that was in her. Her progress had to be reflected back to her so that she could own it, so that our valuing of her efforts could be seen as if a dish she herself had prepared.

Little by little she was able to put more words to her emotions, she could articulate her desires instead of remaining paralyzed: «I want to listen to music», «We can watch video clips», or simply, «Can we go now?». It may perhaps seem a trifle, but for a girl whose survival made continual submission to men necessary, it was not. *In a relationship with a man, Yao Lu had begun to grow, to, dare I say, bloom.*

One day upon my arrival at the Home, I affectionately teased her, and asked, as if I did not know her: «And who are you? Do I know you?». She then gave me a big hug and squeezed me tightly, as she said in smiles «Your little girl!» My position had evolved into that of a solid father figure, but a therapeutic one.

Periodically, she visited her son, who was also progressing and growing. I no longer saw him, as my presence could have been confusing. He was her son, I was not part of that family. We explored her feelings for him. I had accompanied them both during the first eight months of their shared lives. «He's so cute» she said, and I sensed something special in her gaze and smile, or in the way she explained how she would pick him up in her arms. What words would a teenage mother with a life story as hers use?

> It's like happiness... It's the best thing in the world, the best that has ever happened to me, a gift.

I remained silent, affectionately and respectfully, especially after words like those, which echoed and remained suspended in the air. She smiled, but not her distancing smile. She told me: «Heeey!! Don't cry Javier!», yet maybe she said that so as not to cry herself. The emotions expressed that afternoon were moving, I was truly touched. She did let out a few tears, but ones of happiness:

> They're tears of joy ...

Notes

1 In his 1996 article, Bromberg speaks of how essential it is to have a history in order to develop a self and one's mental capacity. He cites Ogden (1989), who warns of the mistake of assuming that patients—*and by extension children, especially children with dissociative dynamics like Yao Lu*—have a sense that their self is continuous over time, in the sense that they feel their present experience is linked to that of their past. (Italics added to the original idea. Ogden, T.H. (1989): *The primitive edge of experience*, Northvale, Basic Books. p.191).

2 Cyrulnik (2007) speaks of a "resilience tutor" as a figure whom these children of battered lives can begin to trust in the projection of a better future, and with whom they can begin to construct the pillars of hope with.

3 E. Ghent (1990) described how, in some cases, a key developmental failure lies in the inability to integrate feelings and impulses to destroy the primary object because they would have been overridden by the parental figures through retaliation, anger, and aggression and—as in the case of Yao Lu—physical and sexual violence. This physical and emotional invasion by the parent, therefore, resulted in difficulty experiencing one's subjectivity as real, perhaps as a result of the paradoxical reactivation of very primitive forms of attachment system due to fear, as P. Fonagy and A. Bateman (2008) suggest. In a situation of trauma, this would hinder the process of mentalization, which would translate into the submission to and the identification with the aggressor, as would have probably occurred with Yao Lu's biological father. She would thus obtain an illusory sense of control over him by being closely identified and submitted to him (if I remain close, submitted, at least I do not get the brunt of his wrath, of the chaos of his emotions). Inherent to this difficulty in separating from the abuser, it is common for the aggressor to become internalized as a dissociated part of the *self*, as a way to *be*, or feel like, a self. This would provide a temporary sense of «relief»—if I suffer I know I exist, or rather, I only exist when I suffer. But now internalized and invisible hatred, instead of being felt as real and outside the self, is transformed into a variety of self-destructive patterns that become the building blocks of the abused identity.

   This construction of the victim's identity remains mostly incomprehensible to the victim, it is the interpersonal air she breathes. As Ghent (1990) pointed out, the effect is therefore that, in order to exist, the impingement of the other becomes necessary, and hence the voluntary masochistic submission is the necessary perversion of surrender—the longed-for security, the cry for affection, the striving for independence, all get silenced (Berliner, 1958). The compulsion to submit (sexually) becomes, in addition to masochistically pleasurable, a form of psychic self-regulation. Although self-destructive, these patterns act to maintain an identity that is otherwise disintegrated in incompatible and tormented parts of her *self*.

4 I never shared the details of the work with Yao Lu with them, and they helped me by showing respect for the privacy of the children I worked with, as well as, indirectly, mine. Maybe that was why I found it so pleasant and comforting to go back home!

5 G. Cecchin (1998) writes about the importance of assuming that we are always vulnerable to reciprocal influence, and that our reactions (even when positively intended) can impede the patient's or family's path towards change; and that is why I suggest we remain humble in the therapeutic relationship and aware of our limitations. S.A. Mitchell (2010) described the therapeutic relationship as involving mutuality, where love and hate emerge, much like what takes place in other intimate relationships. Patients inevitably provoke feelings of love and hate in the therapist! We cannot avoid being affected by them, lest we fall into denial and dissociation to protect ourselves, relying on an illusion of invulnerability that, far from forging a connection, generates distance. Because as therapists, regardless of how well we have worked through our own life, we get emotionally involved with our patients. It is to some degree the fulcrum of treatment (p.128). I would add that in the work with victimized children, perhaps even more.

Referencing Schafer (1976), Mitchell alluded to the «active» character of emotions, pointing to the complexity of emotional life that remains difficult to apprehend. In the «act» of hating or loving, he believed there is a process that performs 'work', which may be difficult to perceive given that love and hate are emotions frequently felt as reactive and spontaneous, but work that has its effect both on the other and on oneself. Whether consciously or unconsciously, loving or hating another person does not usually occur lest we believe there is a good basis for doing so. Therefore the «active» and intentional character of emotions—be it loving or hating or a mixture of both—are not just involuntary occurrences, but take and produce work. From this perspective, emotions could be understood as actions, and re-actions in the construction of more positive relationships. We might «protect» ourselves from the other as 'outside objective observers'. But picking up on children's conscious and unconscious emotions, should not be seen as separate to the intersubjective and «active» character of what we might find ourselves pressured to feel and vice versa. As therapists, we are active participants in the co-constructed process.

6 The Balint groups in Project Sirio were supervision groups moderated by a psychiatrist-therapist, where cases were presented with the group goal of improving the connection, care, and relationship between the therapeutic educator and the specific child. The educators' honesty around emotions and affects that arose in the relationship were fundamental and the quality of the group depended on it.

7 According to T. Ogden (1992) projective identification can be understood as a simultaneous four-part psychological phenomena entailing a primitive mode of object relations, defensive operations, a form of communication, and the delineation of a road to psychic change. For this author, the projection creates a protective distance from the feared and thrust-out aspects of oneself, which for Yao Lu could be the pain, the rage, the feelings of powerlessness at being intruded upon and the lack of privacy in the shanty, as well as her self-identification as an abused girl. In taking these on or experiencing them, in what Mitchell (2010) described as the 'permeability of affects', they take on a communicative function by conveying intelligible and more tangible emotions in the other. As a mode of object relations, by inducing the emotions in the other, one can begin to relate to the intolerable and dissociated lost parts of the *self* within, and start to digest them. Through this lens, by becoming her projection, and through my experience as an invaded and abused therapeutic educator, she could begin to relate, even if only through an attack and rejection, with the different parts of herself, but now external and objectified, induced and embodied in me.

The projection could therefore be understood as a wish for a meeting with the split-off parts of her being, and in this sense it could be an unconscious, intersubjective communication, longing for, and aiming at the integrity of the self. This entailed that projective identification would become, lastly, as Ogden might say, an instrument for psychic change, through which she could process and digest the psychic experience through her relationship with me.

8 Let not teasing humor be confused with sarcasm, for they are very different. Sarcasm intends to inflict pain while teasing humor attempts to leaven the pain of living, to lessen the gap between hope and disappointment, to play with the absurdity of life. Sarcasm sharpens and adds to each of these, its goal being to twist the knife.

Chapter 11

Running out of time:
Where to now?

11.1 In search of a dynamic equilibrium and new technologies

«Being a grown-up», as Yao Lu said that day, was to launch herself into the adventure, to walk through the world of light and darkness, to navigate between the horizons of opportunity and danger without getting shipwrecked, to enjoy life, or crash against the rocks, to construct herself in the reflective shipyards of hope; this was now her path. *Being able to grow despite the adversity and anguish of her memories, to battle them deep inside, to convert them with the help of her therapy and the space of our relationship, to transform them into the narrative of her new story, this was her challenge.* Being a grown-up was to find meaning in her present within the constraints of her past and reach for the future; it was to walk and to smile, to take hold of the responsibility of her life, to be free. But for adolescents, being a grown-up was also to navigate the Internet, a relative novelty at the time!

We set sail on those choppy seas. Obviously, Yao Lu already knew it well and I was no savior opening up a world of opportunities for her behind that blinking cursor. We had listened to music, explored videos, and bid farewell to an email address that had been an important part of her identity. Maybe I could learn something from her. For many, the Internet is the connection to the world ... and there are so many *worlds*!

My initial tendency was to *teach her*. But here I was unknowingly taking the over-inflated position of the stereotypical academic prerogative—«I know more than you, because I am the authority in

DOI: 10.4324/9781003261490-11

the matter»—and I consequently missed out on a lot. Yao Lu smiled and nodded through emotional silences, she seemed to agree with everything I said and followed my lead. How gratifying! I was teaching her so much! But the truth is that I missed it all. I only realized it later on, after Yao Lu went out with that young man she already knew, who groomed her through the online chat, and whom I had suspicions about and had feared. Bound by my own fears and emotions, I had not been able to appreciate hers, the ones I was really interested in. Wishing to protect her, I was unable to hear her. I tried to teach her, but she was unable to communicate. Big parts of her world remained hidden to me, but I had learned that lesson by then.[1]

She disappeared and returned, and after the new lesson, I no longer let the same thing happen again. I apologized for not having been able to pick up on what she was letting me know. I was clearer about my shortcomings and difficulties. And adults make mistakes too. From the domain of reason and *knowledge*, I kept too great a distance from the world of our childhood and its emotions. Maybe that was the reason Peter Pan refused to grow up and return to an adult world, where we have forgotten our dreams, and how to fly.

Next in our shared voyages over the Internet, I became an observant tourist more than a guide. Being prudent about sharing my observations, I was able to see in a way I hadn't, and we took off.

At the Internet café, I invited her to show me what that *chat* thing was all about and how to use it. Soon I was immersed in its frenetic rhythm. Before me, before us, a torrent of hundreds of lonesome Soledades opened up, 709 exactly, all connected with fictional names, in a highly confusing section called «friendship». Our girl was not that uncommon! Each new participant cast out his or her message hoping to find its mooring on a distant relationship. There was no common thread, just a waterfall of brief messages to connect with, disappearing from the screen at a vertiginous rate. It was easy to be flooded by the urgency of despair—«Hi. I want to talk with friends». Yao Lu led the way through that jungle, warning me and showing me who the *undesirable* ones were: those whose messages were too spicy or sexualized amongst the torrent of loneliness.

We spoke about this chat, we had even explored another, and I invited her to reflect on the information she put out about herself. The Internet could be a risky window into the darkness of the world.

She showed me that I could travel to Mexico, Chile, around Spain, and throughout Madrid without getting out of my chair. I let her guide me, and didn't open my mouth. Yao Lu would not have engaged in an inappropriate conversation in front of me. Had it happened, I would have become more active and would have confronted her, or maybe we would have been able to think about what was happening if it involved little risk and it could prevent future dangers online. We were careful about our relationship. I modulated my distance, maintaining a therapeutic posture of not knowing.[2] Shortly after, she asked for my advice, setting the scene for collaborative exchange.

She described to me how she would get overwhelmed by the vertigo of loneliness on the screen, and get snagged on the easy hook of sexual messages, or then would let herself float towards a new encounter.

Windows and invitations to speak in private popped open; some sexually suggestive; others appearing more sincere. I invited her to identify the thieves of innocence with their silken gloves. In short bursts of anger she blocked them one by one. She did not always realize the risks, and I tried to modulate my questions accordingly when the level rose. She connected with a boy who said he was about her age. He showed a friendly interest in her. Our girl was at a loss of what to say about herself, nervously and eagerly asking for my advice. I made small suggestions such as: «I'm nice, cheerful, a good person, a friend to my friends ...». They talked about themselves, about adolescent things. These conversations must have not been too common in her "chat" life, for she closed the other blinking windows as she got into a healthy and meaningful conversation. Her lonely friend responded that she seemed to be an interesting girl. Just as I had been sensing, Yao Lu rapidly typed:

I had a very difficult life before, but now I'm happy.

I'm happy! Well, that sure was gratifying. I was not teaching her anything. She was teaching me! The time came to leave, but we prolonged our work twice. Back in the Home, she spontaneously observed that she was previously incapable of speaking like that on the *chat*. *This was another crucial milestone* on her journey, this time pointed out by her. We braved that path along the real and virtual world again, navigating both surges of anxiety and tranquil seas, dealing with insatiable sexual pirates. But now the route was clearer, the lines and the signs were more easily seen. It was a world better known, under more control.

11.2 Towards a reparative attachment

11.2.1 The secure base

I remember a day when, after I had accompanied her to a job interview, she came out immersed in the anxieties of the moment and began speaking like a tyrant, requesting a prompt return to the Home in her carriage, like an angry queen. She barked at me as she marched towards my car, which we had used that day as a small gesture of support on my behalf, and so we could get there more quickly. I was left perplexed. I walked towards the parking lot feeling the pressure to submit to being a punching bag for her frustrations. I had been waiting for her on the street for an hour and a half! I reached my limit. I told her to stop, severe and serious, this time raising my voice. I never raised my tone, had I gone too far?

She threw her papers to the floor and continued marching on towards the car. I walked up beside her and she apologized. She said she was sorry to have spoken to me like that, and I apologized as well. For a host of reasons, easily guessed at this point, I did my best not to act out my anger; besides, it was just not my style. She confessed, of her own accord, to occasionally needing someone's loud words to nip her angry outburst in the bud, or it would otherwise continue fueling itself.

But my accompaniment was more than momentary, and both humor and the shared sadness we worked through prevailed. Close to two years had gone by. I had been by her side during her pregnancy, and a strong bond had been forged. I had been the recipient and container of her frustrations; I had laughed with her as she learned to trust me and her paranoia towards me waned. I had been shaken by the misadventures of her life; I had felt joy and smiles with each one of her small achievements. She had had so many! We searched for clarity in her confusing and suffocating sexual life. I had gone to look for her in the darkest corners of Madrid, and we had strolled in parks amidst oceans of tears expressing a level of hurt fit for Picasso's Guernica—like when she reclaimed her innocence from the abusive caretaker.

On a day of hard and painful conversations, the words that were perhaps to be the most important ones of our whole process were said. There was *a sort of essence* you could feel in the air, maybe that's what got me to start writing this book—non-transferrable, not exchangeable—which had grown between us. Perhaps even if someone had been there at the time, they would not have perceived it. They were Yao Lu's emotional essences, unique to the care we put into our relationship. And the words came from her not me:

> With you I feel safe. It's as if I've known you my whole life. I'd never spoken with anybody for this long.

Her eighteenth birthday arrived. It brought happiness, angst, and freedom, all wrapped up in great affection. She was there at the Home to celebrate, surrounded by the other adolescents and our team, who shared snippets of her life and story too. After singing *Happy birthday* together, and inviting her to say a few words, our girl shined in the space of her surrogate family. Happy and accompanied, in a wavering voice, she looked out, and yelled:

> That I love you all very muuuuch!

11.2.2 Relationships compared, with whom?

In her progress towards words, Yao Lu had shared her fears, her sadness, her laughter, and her hopes with me. Sometimes she shared them as soon as I arrived, other times she hurried me along for us to reach our accustomed space for conversation, so she could tell me there. One of those days, she timidly told me she had met a boy.

I responded cautiously; on one hand she had a very hard time sharing this type of experience while she was living it; on the other hand I ran the risk of being experienced as judgmental (like her mother), which would end up making her feel like she didn't want to speak. This had happened to me on occasion. For instance, when she had told me of questionable friendships in her different previous residential facilities, if I dared criticize them, I inadvertently turned her into the passive object of my critique. At the end of the day, she would say herself that they might not have been the best company, that they had problems like her, but they were the ones who were there. Could they be advisable traveling companions for Yao Lu? If these young companions could not to be recommended, neither could she. They were all in similar situations. Therefore, contrary to my intention, I forged an impossible situation for her. The implicit message was that she herself could not be a good friend, or that other people would see her as unworthy of their friendship. There was no way other than she explore and discover, and make these judgments on her own.

Yao Lu wanted friendships. She had searched for them everywhere, including in the torrent of Lonelinesses (Soledades) on the Internet chat. She explained how she had approached a boy, and despite being painfully shy, had shaken his hand, without jumping into long-winded explanations of her life as she used to, «I was cautious». She introduced herself, they spoke and he invited her out to dance a few days later. Our girl felt flattered and respected by him. She had not told anyone yet when she revealed it to me. Given my accepting attitude, she spoke freely not only of her excitement, but also of feeling like a responsible adult, as her ownership and freedom in life grew. She felt proud and I have to say, I felt proud of her too.

I had strolled through shopping malls with Yao Lu, letting her browse the stores on her own to look at clothes. We would stop to observe the groups of kids her age. It sometimes seemed that she looked at them as if they were from another planet, a world she longed for with much curiosity.

She met another boy during those weeks, this time through the *chat*. With a twinkle in her eyes, she told me they were the same age, and that he liked to talk. The story she then told me revealed the possibility that she was relating to men in a new way. Apparently, he reminded her of me! What would I be like to Yao Lu? There was the risk of my becoming narcissistically preoccupied, unconsciously pressuring her to gratify me through her flattery, at least indirectly. But it was not my job to be liked, nor was it her job to make me feel good. My job was to be aware of this risk and work on it from within, so it would not be pathologically reproduced in our relationship.[3] "What I was like" resided in her experience of our relationship. «He's like you … but more like a kid!», and she laughed as she explained that he was a serene and respectful conversationalist.

In her history, some boys had occasionally been respectful of her, but most others acted quite the opposite. Our girl began to be able to leave or to put a stop to those relations when she so wished, thus breaking the chains of her traumatic past. I conveyed that she showed strength in doing so. Yao Lu had been able to deal with quite a lot in her life, and I was certain she could go on moving forwards. She lit up when she heard it—«Yea, I'm working hard and moving down the right path...»—as if she were saying: «I'm managing well and feel it to be true, thank you». I was proud of each and every one of her steps forward, her steps, not mine, and that is what I tried to convey on a daily basis. The crises she was immersed in at times could now be seen as a necessary part of her progress. Are they not for everyone? The only difference was the serious danger she had put herself in.

Yao Lu wanted to change, she wanted to rebuild her life and she wanted to be happy. For that matter, she wanted to prove to everybody that she could do it. She wanted it so much—«I want to prove it to myself»—that, after a long silence, she carefully chose her words:

> That I'm worth it...

Yao Lu was a *survivor*, not a mere *victim, as I had tried to convey to her.* The word survivor includes having been a victim, but it also entails a very different meaning. Rebuilt from her wounds and her subsequent setbacks, her survival was now converted into successful progress. Yao Lu was moving forward.[4]

The relationship with her mother was also improving, though with sporadic derailments that could be likened to the course of a confusing tango. Since our girl no longer acted out her anger as much, her mother could thus come closer in a gradual reconnection. Both of them could share and grow in their positive experiences together. Our girl began to feel more accompanied by her mother, and the mother, occasionally, by her daughter.

11.2.3 Boyfriend rehearsals

Her relationship with the boy she had met was growing. She said she was getting to know him judiciously. She felt taken care of by him and received his calls to wish her happy holidays, and to inquire as to how she was doing. What a novelty for our girl-mother-teen who had previously known only the indifference of the toxic masculine world! She told me how his words took care of her, encouraged her to keep moving forwards. They went to the movies and to dinner. «I have like a tingling feeling», she said pointing at her stomach and smiling happily.

Love must have been so strange for a girl who perhaps had never received it until then. In fact, it even roused doubts in some of the colleagues on our team. What is love? An age-old question. It might just be an intangible essence, an experience people hope to share. I leave the rest to poets.

Notes

1 She moved between submission and surrender (Ghent, E. 1990) in our relationship, surrender being a mutual surrender of intersubjective awareness, in a complex therapeutic process. We were inextricably woven together as we moved through the different states and emotions of our girl-teenager-mother, and there was a subtle echo of the relational trauma of her past, but we also created/surrendered to a relational way of being, which Benjamin (2004) calls «thirdness». This field is one where both members of the relationship can be seen at once, allowing them to gradually evolve into subject-to-subject modes of relating, from subject-to-object (Ringstrom, 2007) ones. From objects to be «used» we would transform the relationship, co-construct it (Ogden, 1992; also in Ringstrom, 2007) into a mutual encounter, where we would both learn from each other and change each other.

2 Yao Lu was the expert in that world, just as she was in her own, and I had never ceased to be solely a guest. H. Anderson & H. Goolishian (1992) wrote about this therapeutic posture in a very clarifying way, in their article «The client is the expert: a not-knowing approach to therapy».

3 J. Barudy and M. Dantagnan (2005) make note of this in their book *Los buenos tratos a la infancia*. (The title could likely be translated as: Good treatment in childhood).

4 Being a «survivor» helped with the integration of the alienated parts of her *self*, the «not-me's» that were so terrifying and difficult to identify (Sullivan 1953), into a more coherent and less pain-ridden experience, less fragmented by trauma that she had wanted to rid herself of only to re-find it so many times. The fact that I had been able to see those different parts of her, hold them in their emotional-relational complexity, mentalize them (Fonagy, 1991; Fonagy & Bateman, 2008; Fonagy &

Target, 2006; Slade, 2006) without rejecting them, without re-dissociating them, but to explore them in a context of care, a context co-created in the surrender of us both—perhaps all this had also managed to help her initiate a more stable internal dialogue between her self-states and to establish the healthy illusion of a more coherent, less dispersed, more unitary sense of self (Bromberg, 1996, 2003). Less dominated by her anxieties, more capable of thinking reflectively (*reflective functioning*) (Slade, A., 2006), she had become less afraid to think about thinking (Fonagy, 1991) as she felt, decided, and thought without dissociating as much.

Chapter 12

Individuation and autonomy

12.1 Separation, attachment, and time to stop

Yao Lu, once more, disappeared. I did not see her in our Home again. This departure was different though. It had nothing to do with her previous flights. Our girl moved on to a shared and planned life with *her boyfriend*.

The radical break unnerved me, but she took care to keep us informed of her wellbeing by phone, a shift that carried important implicit meanings. I reflected on her treatment to see if and how it fit her life process.

The New Year had come and gone, and I gave our girl space. After waiting a few more days, I went over to where they lived and called on her. In humor, *I reprimanded* her for not being there at my last scheduled visit to the Home. We laughed together and the atmosphere was relaxed. I invited her to meet, since we had not wished each other a happy New Year, and I admit that I also wanted to assess her new situation.

She expressed concern that I might want to take her back to the Home. I calmly let her know I was only coming to visit her and, as she already knew, that she could decide to return if she wished, that it was her choice. *Our girl had come of age*, and she had continued living with us voluntarily, until an adequate place could be found for her.

Shortly thereafter, we got together to wish each other a happy New Year, with an affectionate hug. She seemed well, hopeful, and calm, and she compared old experiences with her present. They had a shower with hot water and it was something she felt was important, compared to still recent experiences in Madrid's fourth world!

DOI: 10.4324/9781003261490-12

Proud, and perhaps searching for validation from me, she said:

> I now live with my partner.

I cautiously inquired about her situation and what she felt about it. I could not lean prematurely in any direction yet. What if it did not work out? Would she blame me? Worse still, would I have become a rival in her relationship? Maybe I too had a hard time separating. Yao Lu was building a new bond, and if it was positive and made her grow, I had to begin to fade out.

She knew she was loved by us, she felt affection from the team, but as she said, «I want my own life». How normal!

I still feared that this could be a new flight and an emotional escape to the illusory shelter of a new partner, as a way to avoid continuing to work through her sorrows in the fiction of a new autonomy.[1] Even if that were the case, who was I to decide for her? Yao Lu told me about a positive and reparative departure from the Home, and although I thought she had high expectations for her partner to live up to, she seemed happy. My confidence was not wholehearted and I did feel a hint of fear, but she was right: it was her life and it was time for me to say goodbye.

Still a little skeptical, I asked if she would be living his life or hers. But I was able to confirm that by now our little girl had grown and matured, when she answered leaving me astonished: «Ours!». What more could I say?

At times, like caring parents, those of us who work with adolescents with such serious problems find it hard to let go and say goodbye. Prey to our own fears, we run the risk of hindering the flight of those who are, precisely, learning to fly with our help. We fear failure and long for the certainty of their wellbeing. Because of our fears and anxieties, we make it difficult for them to separate.

I too had grown a great deal during this time. The moment may have taken me by surprise, but I knew that it was time to end our walks strewn with difficult experiences and uncertain situations. Yao Lu had started to distance herself from me on her own initiative— another success to check off her bucket list—and our relationship began to fade, but not our bond. This would remain, and would become stronger with this step towards freedom that I had helped foster. However far she would fly, our bond would go with her as a referential pillar.

Her partner, a few years younger than I was at the time (late twenties), could see me as a rival and, I could unwillingly become a source of unnecessary conflict between them. Yao Lu would maintain a psychotherapeutic space with our psychiatrist and director, but my time of accompanying her had come to its end. It was with all of this in my mind that I approached our work those days. I still encouraged reflection on her actions, for she was intermittently missing her treatment sessions, and she had also missed the latest visitation with her son. She considered the possible and definitive reunion with him as very distant, but I knew she wanted to stay in touch with him. There was a lot for her to think about, and so she did. She wanted to continue in therapy to sort out her life. After all, we had been bastions of support and help, and she would still have much to work on in the future, but our time of work together with me was running out.

We considered it problematic to continue with visits, so we invited her to request them if she so wished. Although she did not seem convinced that we should see each other, perhaps perceiving the possible uneasiness of her partner, we spoke on the phone many times. She excitedly told me about her adventures of the moment— «I'm buying groceries, Javier!»—, a novelty in Yao Lu's young adult life, as the cashier's machines could be overheard in the background ringing up the items. On another call, not able to contain her excitement, she cheerfully told me that she had gone to register to vote in her new neighborhood.

I was available by phone, and so we worked through our termination.

The time had come for her to bloom, and I remembered a conversation from months before. After offering a narrative full of success and as we attended to her tears and her smiles, she told me: «It's just that sometimes I sink...». I responded:

Sometimes you have to sink to grow ... like seeds that sink into the ground, to then become a flower ... What flower would you want to be, Yao Lu?
—A rose.

In a firm and affectionate whisper, I pointed out: «Good Yao Lu, but not too many thorns, don't prick yourself so much», and our girl blossomed in wide smiles.

So long Yao Lu, so long.

Note

1 On the process of differentiation of the self and the dynamics of family systems, and the autonomy and pseudo-autonomy of its members, I recommend the book by M. Bowen (1978), which accompanied me over the course of our young girl's process.

Conclusions?

C.1

I am not too sure what I should write here. I am not too sure I even have the tools to comment and to capture the work we shared. Perhaps, on the other hand, it is also hard because doing so somehow, is saying goodbye, and in saying goodbye it is now me who is being left.

Yao Lu accompanied me for nearly three and a half years—or was it me that accompanied her? Truth is, it's hard to say and the lines are blurry. There have been so many experiences that I do not even know if I have written about the right ones. What I do know is that she is with me. She is a reference and an experiential memento in my daily work, and I imagine that, having been my most important training case, perhaps she will accompany me without being there, for a long time more. I just hope I reached her enough to have been a positive influence in her life and that she is now able to feel more free, wherever she may go.

Maybe when I miss her, it shows that the work was good, because a positive attachment must be mutual in nature. It cannot exist otherwise. It has to be constructed in a positively charged interpersonal space where both grow through their shared experiences. It must also be a place to reencounter oneself. If not, there is a risk of forging symbiotic, toxic, or mutually dependent bonds. The work was with and for our girl-mother Yao Lu, a girl who made her way in the world from a place far away. And as I worked with this girl, I also somehow worked with my own inner child. I had a great time! I suffered too.

I understand that she had to fly away, and perhaps the goal of the work had been to allow it in the end, like a good father does. I will be with Yao Lu in her memories, of that I am sure, and no matter how far away she might be, I will surface in her reminiscences of experiences we shared, just as she will with me. The therapeutic accompaniment was not so much about guiding, but about being and becoming, about rediscovery, about frustrating the impossible, and about allowing for what was, to grow, to create something new, a bond, and to explore the world in freedom. That was the essence.

Can I summarize this? The truth is I'm not too sure. I must own my incompetence yet again, in order to continue learning how to turn on the lights of small hopes that may brighten the nights of children. By doing this, I myself light up. If I am pressed for clarifications and technique, I will say with Saint-Exupéry: «And now here is my secret, a very simple secret: It is only with the heart that one can see rightly; what is essential is invisible to the eye».

«What is essential is invisible to the eye … ».

Javier

Addendum: Five years from the report filed against Marcelo by Javier and Yao Lu's mother, Javier was summoned to give a deposition before the trial. He came from New York to provide his statement and support his little girl in that drawn out battle against the abuse. He felt he had to do so, both for personal and professional reasons. He was then working as an adolescent and family therapist in the state of New York.

C.2

Beloved girl of ours, Yao Lu, though you are no longer a girl since many years have passed since this story of yours and ours, told here in this book so we can all think and learn.

—Do you remember Javier?
—Of course!!
—Do you think he was able to help you then, or helped you in something, in this shared work?
   [Many seconds of silence, more silence]
—He helped me be more free.

After this thoughtful, clear and concise declaration by our protagonist, a seal of approval from my perspective as director of the Project that our long and shared work had been worth while, it seems necessary, in finishing up, to add three additional notes, pointing to the importance of each one of these themes, which will need further work and research, and which are embedded throughout our book as a whole. Our tale, grounded in the reality in which we work, will have an even more open ending, or if possible, no end:

1. Intersubjectivity: a specifically human and mature relationship is shown here. In this narrative, two subjectivities meet, share life as they journey through their development, growth, and splendor, with boundaries.
2. The knowledge of the genesis and development of moral conscience: this is initiated in the first and second year of the life of the child—provided the attachment with the mother takes place and the rearing is adequate—with its necessary and indispensable qualities of reciprocity and empathy. It might be understood better, or perhaps in a new light, with an understanding of this case.
3. Borderline personality disorder: a pathology that afflicts mostly adolescents and young adults, manifests itself with increasing force in psychiatric consulting rooms across the board, and it presents its key symptoms as a great instability in interpersonal relationships, in self-image and in affectivity, as well as a notorious impulsivity. This disorder, which is accompanied by severe and secondary difficulties in daily life, could be better understood upon careful attentive reading of our story.

Many professionals, colleagues, and other people who know of our Project, ask us and wonder about the success or failure of our work with the children.

Is Yao Lu's life now a success? What is she up to? What does she do for a living? Does she still hold down a job? Have a partner?

It is then, and with increasing frequency, that the complex, mythical, brilliant figure of Marilyn Monroe comes to our minds. Her life was so similar to that of Yao Lu's, at least in their first two decades. In much the same way, more than 50 years since her disappearance: she is a shining star, iconic, successful, an enormously attractive person to many; a vital failure, consumed by loneliness and impotence, a victim, to others.

With these final lines, silence and reflection are called for—or the ever so crucial process of mentalization, which we worked on with Yao Lu, as we do with all of our children—so that the readers may thus extract their own conclusions, the ones that might truly matter.

María Eugenia

C.3

On this cold winter morning, after years have passed since this story, Yao Lu brings her little notepad with «the homework done» on it, and it says:

This is what I think now, of my life after reading this book closely, with you, dear María Eugenia. I have laughed reading some things, I have relived many moments. Poor Javier, the things he had to go through at times! I have also felt sorrow. It has made me think and remember.

I think that I have matured a lot since then. I see that I did many silly things before, I thought little. But loneliness, to feel lonely, that's very hard, it's really tough. In life you need to be hugged, you need people to treat you with affection, to believe in you, and keep you in mind, to be important to someone.

Could I say something to other young people or adolescents, in situations similar to mine?

- Whatever you do wrong, think about it. Think about what you are going to do so later you don't have so much to regret.
- To the people that love you, ask them for help. Never listen to people who aren't good for you.
- Never let yourself be tricked by anyone, especially by the ones who hurt you.
- Always do things that feel right to you; not for others, not just to please someone else.
- Leave the things that harm you and never think of taking your life.
- For those who are close to you, for those who love you, let yourself be helped; and not by the people that take advantage of you and treat you like trash.

- Each day you have to try to be more positive and think of fixing things and the problems, of getting past your difficulties. And keep moving forwards, slightly better each day.
- Never give up. Life will gift you with the most beautiful things when you least expect it.
- And always be very patient.

Yao Lu

Bibliography

Abad, M. (2001). «El abuso sexual. Comentario sobre un caso clínico». *Aperturas Psicoanalíticas, Revista Internacional de Psicoanálisis*, 31. Open access in: www.aperturas.org. [Commentary on the article by Inji, R. (2001): «Countertransference, enactment and sexual abuse», *Journal of Child Psychotherapy,* 27, 285–301. 10.1080/00754170110087568].

Abrams, J. (1990). «Eternal youth and narcissism: The child's dilemma». In J. Abrams (Ed.), *Reclaiming the Inner Child* (p. 117). Los Angeles, CA: Jeremy P. Tarcher.

Ackerman, N. W. (1962). Family psychotherapy and psychoanalysis: The implications of difference. *Family Process*, 1(1), 30–43. 10.1111/j.1545-5300.1962.00030.x.

Altman, N. (2008). «From fathering daughters to doddering father». *Psychoanalytic Inquiry*, 28, 92–105. 10.1080/07351690701787135.

Anderson, H., & Goolishian, H. (1992). The client is the expert: A not-knowing approach to therapy. In S. McNamee & K. Gergen, (Eds.), *Social Construction and the Therapeutic Process* (pp. 25–39). Newbury Park, CA: Sage Publications.

Bahrick, L. E., & Watson, J. S. (1985). Detection of intermodal proprioceptive–Visual contingency as a potential basis of self-perception in infancy. *Developmental Psychology*, 21(6), 963–973. https://doi.org/10.1037/0012-1649.21.6.963.

Barrie, J. M. (1911). *Peter and Wendy*. New York: Charles Scribners Sons. [Edited, published and later known as *Peter Pan*].

Barudy, J., & Dantagnan, M. (2005). *Los Buenos Tratos a la Infancia; Parentalidad, Apego y Resiliencia*. Barcelona: Editorial Gedisa.

Bateson, G., Jackson, D., Haley, J., & Weakland, J. (1956). «Toward a theory of schizophrenia». In C. Sluzki & D. Ranson (Eds.) (1976), *Double*

Bind, The Foundation of the Communicational Approach to the Family (pp. 3–22). New York: Grune & Stratton. 10.1002/bs.3830010402.

Bebee, B., & Lachman, F. (1996). «The three principles of salience in the organization of the patient-analyst interaction». *Psychoanalytic Psychology*, 13, 1–22. 10.1037/h0079635.

Bebee, B., & Lachman, F. (1998). «Co-constructing inner and relational processes: Self and mutual regulation in infant research and adult treatment». *Psychoanalytic Psychology*, 15, 480–516. 10.1037/0736-9735.15.4.480.

Benjamin, J. (2004). «Beyond doer and done-to: An intersubjective view of thirdness». *Psychoanal Quart*, 73, 5–46. 10.1002/j.2167-4086.2004.tb00151.x.

Benjamin, J. (2009). «Psychoanalytic controversies. A relational psychoanalysis perspective on the necessity of acknowledging failure in order to restore the facilitating and containing features of the intersubjective relationship (the shared third)». *International Journal of Psychoanalysis*, 90, 441–450. 10.1111/j.1745-8315.2009.00163.x.

Berger, P., & Luckmann, T. (1991). *The Social Construction of Reality*. London: Penguin Books.

Berliner, B. B. (1958). «The role of object relations in moral masochism». *Psychoanalytic Quarterly*, 27, 38–56. DOI: 10.1080/21674086.1958.11926077.

Berne, E. (1975). *Games People Play; The Psychology of Human Relationships*. London: Penguin Books. 10.1192/S0007125000219247.

Bernier, A., & Meins, E. (2008). A threshold approach to understanding the origins of attachment disorganization. *Developmental Psychology*, 44(4), 969–982. 10.1037/0012-1649.44.4.969.

Bettelheim, B. (2010). *The Uses of Enchantment: The Meaning and Importance of Fairy Tales*. New York: Vintage Books.

Bion, W. R. (1990). *Brazilian Lectures*. London: Karnac Books.

Bornstein, M. H., & Sigman, M. (1986). Continuity in mental development from infancy. *Child Development*, 57, 251–274. 10.2307/1130581.

Boston Change Process Study Group (2018). Moving through and being moved by: Embodiment in development and in the therapeutic relationship. *Contemporary Psychoanalysis*, 54(2), 299–321. 10.1080/00107530.2018.1456841.

Bowen, M. (1978). *Family Therapy in Clinical Practice*. New York: Jason Aronson.

Bowlby, J. (1979). *The Making and Breaking of Affectional Bonds*. London: Tavistock Publications.

Bowlby, J. (1988). *A Secure Base: Parent-Child Attachment and Healthy Human Development*. New York: Basic Books.

Bromberg, P. (1996). «Standing in the spaces: The multiplicity of self and the psychoanalytic relationship». *Contemporary Psychoanalysis*, 32, 509–535. 10.1080/00107530.1996.10746334.

Bromberg, P. (2003). «Something wicked this way comes: Trauma, dissociation, and conflict: The space where psychoanalysis, cognitive science and neuroscience overlap». *Psychoanalytic Psychology*, 20, 558–574. 10.1 037/0736-9735.20.3.558.

Bromberg, P. (2008). «Shrinking the tsunami. Affect regulation, dissociation, and the shadow of the flood». *Contemporary Psychoanalysis*, 44, 329–350. 10.1080/00107530.2008.10745961.

Buber, M. (1958). *I and Thou*. New York: Scribner's.

Bucay, J. (2013). *Let Me Tell You a Story: Tales along the Road to Happiness* (Trans. by L. Dillman). New York: Europa Editions. [Original published in Spanish (2002): *Déjame que te cuente: Los cuentos que me enseñaron a vivir*, Barcelona, RBA Libros].

Caflisch, J. (2012). «Submission and surrender: The case of Fatima». *Contemporary Psychoanalysis*, 48, 29–53. 10.1080/00107530.2012.10746488.

Carlson, E. (1998). A prospective longitudinal study of attachment disorganization/disorientation. *Child Development*, 69(4), 1107–1128. 10.1111/j. 1467-8624.1998.tb06163.x.

Carlson, V., Cicchetti, D., Barnett, D., & Braunwald, K. (1989). Disorganized/ disoriented attachment relationships in maltreated infants. *Developmental Psychology*, 25(4), 525–531. 10.1037/0012-1649.25.4.525.

Cecchin, G. (1998). «Sistemas terapéuticos y terapeutas». In M. Elkaïm (Ed.), *La terapia familiar en transformación* (pp. 63–66). Barcelona: Paidós Ibérica. [Unavailable in English to the authors' knowledge. Original compilation published in French as: *Le thérapie familiale en changement*].

Cyr, C., Euser, E., Bakermans-Kranenburg, M., & Van Ijzendoorn, M. (2010). Attachment security and disorganization in maltreating and high-risk families: A series of meta-analyses. *Development and Psychopathology*, 22(1), 87–108. 10.1017/S0954579409990289.

Cyrulnik, B. (2007). *Talking of Love on the Edge of a Precipice* (Trans. by D. Macey). London: Allen Lane-Penguin Books. [First published in French as *Parler d'Amour au bord de gouffre*, 2005].

De Waal, F. (2006). *Primates and Philosophers: How Morality Evolved* (S. Macedo & J. Ober, Eds.). Princeton, NJ: Princeton University Press.

Dickens, C. (1921). *A Tale of Two Cities*. Nueva York: Cosmopolitan Book Corporation.

Eisold, B. (2012). «The implications of family expectations, historical trauma, and prejudice in psychoanalytic psychotherapy with naturalized and first-generation Chinese Americans». *Contemporary Psychoanalysis*, 48, 238–266. 10.1080/00107530.2012.10746500.

Elkaïm, M. (1997). *If You Love Me, Don't Love Me: Undoing Reciprocal Double Binds and Other Methods of Change in Couple & Family Therapy* (Trans. by H. Chubb). New York: Jason Aronson. [First published in French as: *Si tu m'aimes, ne m'aime pas. Approche systémique et psychothérapie.* Editions du Seuil, Paris, 1989].

Emde, R. N., Biringen, Z., Clyman, R. B., & Oppenheim, D. (1991). The moral self of infancy: Affective core and procedural knowledge. *Developmental Review*, 11, 251–270. 10.1016/0273-2297(91)90013-E.

Erikson, E. H. (1963). *Childhood and Society.* New York: W.W. Norton.

Eskelinen de Folch, T. (1988). «Communication and containing in child analysis: Towards terminability». *International Journal of Psycho-Analysis*, 69, 105–112.

Felitti, V. J., Anda, R. F., Nordenberg, D., Williamson, D. F., Spitz, A. M., Edwards, V., Koss, M. P., & Marks, J. S. (1998). Relationship of childhood abuse and household dysfunction to many of the leading causes of death in adults: The Adverse Childhood Experiences (ACE) Study. *American Journal of Preventive Medicine*, 14(4), 245–258. 10.1016/S0749-3797(98)00017-8.

Ferenczi, S. (1949). «The confusion of the tongues between the adults and the child —(The language of tenderness and of passion)». *International Journal of Psycho- Analysis*, 30, 225–230.

Foerster, H., & Müller, A. (2008). «Computing a reality. Heinz von Foerster's lecture at the A.U.M Conference in 1973. Edited by Albert Müller». *Constructivist Foundations*, 4(1), 62–69.

Fogel, A. (1992). «Movement and communication in human infancy: The social dynamics of development». *Human Movement Science*, 11, 387–423. https://doi.org/10.1016/0167-9457(92)90021-3.

Fonagy, P. (1991). «Thinking about thinking: Some clinical and theoretical considerations in the treatment of a borderline patient». *International Journal of Psycho-Analysis*, 72, 639–656.

Fonagy, P., & Bateman, A. (2008). «The development of borderline personality disorder. A mentalizing model». *Journal of Personality Disorders*, 22, 4–21. 10.1521/pedi.2008.22.1.4.

Fonagy, P., Gergely, G., Jurist, E., & Target, M. (2002). *Affect Regulation, Mentalization, and the Development of the self.* New York: Other Press.

Fonagy, P., & Target, M. (2006). «The mentalization focused approach to self pathology». *Journal of Personality Disorders*, 20, 544–576. 10.1521/pedi.2006.20.6.544.

Frankl, V. E. (1962). *Man's Search for Meaning: An Introduction to Logotherapy*. Boston: Beacon Press.

Frankl, V. E. (1968). *Psychotherapy and Existentialism: Selected Papers on Logotherapy*. New York: Simon & Schuster.

Freud, A., & Burlingham, D. T. (1973). *Infants without Families: Reports on the Hampstead Nurseries, 1939–1945*. New York: International Universities Press.

Fuentes, J. (1983). «El sistema, la comunicación y la familia». In T. Suárez & C. F. Rojero (dir). *Paradigma sistémico y terapia de familia*, Madrid: Asociación Española de Neuropsiquiatría.

Gedaly, R. L. & Leerkes, M. E. (2016) The role of sociodemographic risk and maternal behavior in the prediction of infant attachment disorganization. *Attachment & Human Development*, 18(6), 554–569. 10.1 080/14616734.2016.1213306.

Gergely G., & Watson J. S. (1996). «The social biofeedback model of parent affect mirroring». *International Journal of Psycho-Analysis*, 77, 1181–1212.

Ghent, E. (1990). «Masochism, submission, surrender-massochism as a perversion of surrender». *Contemporary Psychoanalysis*, 26, 108–136. 10.1 080/00107530.1990.10746643.

Goffman, E. (1986). *Stigma: Notes on the Management of Spoiled Identity*. New York: Touchstone.

Green, A. H. (1980). *Child Maltreatment*. New York: Jason Aronson.

Grossmark, R. (2016). «Psychoanalytic companioning». *Psychoanalytic Dialogues*, 26, 698–712. 10.1080/10481885.2016.1235447.

Herrero, M. E. (2009). «El trastorno de la vinculación en niños y adolescentes y los estados predelirantes». *Congreso Interpsiquis. Psiquiatria.com, 13(2)*. http://psiqu.com/1-6448.

Jaffe, J., Beebe, B., Feldstein, S., Crown, C., & Jasnow, M. (2001). «Rhythms of dialogues in infancy: coordinated timing in development». *Monographs of the Society for Research in Child Development*, 66(2), 1–149.

Karoly, L., Kilburn, M., & Cannon, J. (2005). *Early Childhood Interventions: Proven Results, Future Promise*. Santa Monica, CA; Arlington, VA; Pittsburgh, PA: RAND Corporation. 10.7249/MG341.

Kernberg, P. F., Weiner, A. S., & Bardenstein, K. K. (2000). *Personality Disorders in Children and Adolescents*. New York: Basic Books.

Knudson-Martin, C., & Mahoney, A. R. (1999). «Beyond different worlds: A "Postgender" approach to relational development». *Family Process*, 38, 325–340. 10.1111/j.1545-5300.1999.00325.x.

Kohlberg, L. (1981). *Essays on Moral Development, Vol. I: The Philosophy of Moral Development*. San Francisco, CA: Harper & Row.

Laing, R. D. (1965). «Mystification, confusion, and conflict». In C. Sluzki & D. Ranson (Eds.), *Double Bind, The Foundation of the Communicational Approach to the Family* (pp. 199–218). New York: Grune & Stratton.

Laing, R. D. (1968). *The Politics of Experience*. New York: Ballantine Books.

Lerner, H. G. (1989). *The Dance of Anger*. New York: Perennial Library, Harper & Row.

Levin, J. (1993). *Slings and Arrows: Narcissistic Injury and Its Treatment*. Northvale, NJ: Jason Aronson.

Linares, J. L. (1996). *Identidad y Narrativa*. Barcelona: Paidos Ibérica, S.A.

Lyons-Ruth, K. (2003). Dissociation and the parent-infant dialogue: A longitudinal perspective from attachment research. *Journal of the American Psychoanalytic Association*, 51, 883–911. 10.1177/00030651030510031501.

Lyon-Ruth, K., Bruschweiler-Stern, N., Harrison, A. M., Morgan, A. C., Nahum, J. P., Sander, L., Stern, D. N. Y., & Tronick, E. Z. (1998). «Implicit relational knowing: Its role in development and psychoanalytic treatment». *Infant Mental Health Journal*, 19, 282–289. https://doi.org/1 0.1002/(SICI)1097-0355(199823)19:3<282::AID-IMHJ3>3.0.CO;2-O.

Lyons-Ruth, K., & Jacobvitz, D. (2016). Attachment disorganization: Genetic factors, parenting contexts, and developmental transformation from infancy to adulthood. In J. Cassidy & P. Shaver (Eds.), *Handbook of Attachment: Theory, Research, and Clinical Applications* (3rd ed., pp. 667–696). New York: Guilford Press.

Marina, J. (2006). *Anatomía del miedo; un tratado sobre la valentía*. Barcelona: Anagrama.

May, R. (1953). *Man's Search for Himself*. New York: W.W. Norton.

Mead, M. (1968). «Cybernetics of cybernetics». In H. Von Foerster, J. White, & J. Russell (comp.). *Purposive Systems*, New York: Spartan Books.

Miller, A. (1981). *The Drama of the Gifted Child. The Search for the True Self*. New York: Basic Books.

Mitchell, S. A. (2010). *Relationality: From Attachment to Intersubjectivity*. New York: Routledge Mental Health. 10.4324/9781315803289.

Moreno, Z. T. (1978). The function of the auxiliary ego in psychodrama with special reference to psychotic patients. *Group Psychotherapy, Psychodrama & Sociometry*, 31, 163–166.

Múgica, J. (2006). «Adopción y abandono, las dos caras de una misma realidad». *Revista Mosaico*, June, n° 35, Federación Española de Asociaciones de Terapia Familiar.

Neuburger, R. (1997). *La familia dolorosa; mito y terapias familiares*. Barcelona: Editorial Herder. [First published in French as Le Mythe Familial, 1995].

Nhat Hanh, T. (2001). *Calming the Fearful Mind. A Zen Response to Terrorism*. Berkeley, CA: Paralax Press.

Normandin, L., Ensink, K., Yeomans, F. E., Kernberg, O. F. (2014). «Transference- focused psychotherapy for personality disorders in adolescence». In C. Sharp & J. L. Tackett (Eds.), *Handbook of Borderline Personality Disorder in Children and Adolescents* (pp. 333–359). New York: Springer. 10.1007/978-1-4939-0591-1_22.

Ogden, T. H. (1992). *Projective Identification and Psychotherapeutic Technique*. London: Karnac Books.

Papousek, H. (1981). The common in the uncommon child. In M. Lewis & L. Rosenblum (Eds.), *The Uncommon Child* (pp. 317–328). New York: Plenum.

Peck, S. M. (1990). «Love and the fear of abandonment». In J. Abrams (Ed.), *Reclaiming the Inner Child* (pp. 104–105). Los Angeles, CA: Jeremy P. Tarcher.

Picasso, P. (1937). *Guernica [oil on canvas]*. Madrid, Spain: Museo Nacional Centro de Arte Reina Sofía.

Ringstrom, P. A. (2007). «Scenes that write themselves: Improvisational moments in relational psychoanalysis». *Psychoanalytic Dialogues, 17*, 69–99. 10.1080/10481880701301303.

Roland, A. (1996). «The influence of culture on the self and selfobject relationships: An Asian-north American comparison». *Psychoanalytic Dialogues: The International Journal of Relational Perspectives, 6*(4), 461–475. 10.1080/10481889609539131.

Saint-Exupéry, A. (1971). *The Little Prince* (Trans. by K. Woods) New York: Harcourt Brace Jovanovich.

Schafer, R. (1976). *A New Language for Psychoanalysis*. New Haven, CT: Yale University Press.

Sebastián, J. (2000). «Género, salud y psicoterapia». In M. J. Carrasco & A. García-Mina (Eds.), *Género y psicoterapia* (pp. 11–36). Madrid: Publications from the Universidad Pontificia of Comillas.

Slade, A. (2006). «Reflective parenting programs: Theory and development». *Psychoanalytic Inquiry, 26*, 640–657. 10.1080/07351690701310698

Sonntag, M. (2007). «The bonds of hate». *Studies in Gender and Sexuality, 8*, 97–112.

Spitz, R. A. (1945). «Hospitalism: An inquiry into the genesis of psychiatric conditions in early childhood». *Psychoanalytic Study of the Child, 1*, 53–74. 10.1080/00797308.1945.11823126.

Sroufe, L. A. (2005). Attachment and development: A prospective, longitudinal study from birth to adulthood. *Attachment & Human Development, 7*(4), 349–367. 10.1080/14616730500365928.

Stern, D. (1985). *The Interpersonal World of the Infant*. New York: Basic Books.

Stern, D. (1995). *The Motherhood Constellation*. New York: Basic Books.

Sullivan, H. S. (1953). *The Interpersonal Theory of Psychiatry*. New York: W.W. Norton.

Trefler, D. (2009). Quality is free: A cost-benefit analysis of early child development initiatives. *Paediatrics & Child Health*, 14(10), 681–684. 10.1 093/pch/14.10.681.

Vaillant, M. (2004). «Reciclaje de la violencia y capacidad de resiliencia: la hipótesis transicional en la reparación». In B. Cyrulnik, S. Tomkiewicz, T. Guénard, & others. *El realismo de la esperanza; testimonios de experiencias profesionales en torno a la resiliencia*. Barcelona: Editorial Gedisa.

Vanistendael, S. (2004). «Humor y resiliencia: La sonrisa que da vida». In B. Cyrulnik, S. Tomkiewicz, T. Guénard, & others. *El realismo de la esperanza; testimonies de experiencias profesionales en torno a la resiliencia*. Barcelona: Editorial Gedisa.

Von Foerster, H. (1973). «Cybernetic of cybernetics (physiology of revolution)». *The Cybernetitian*, 3, 30–32.

Watzlawick, P., Bavelas, J. B., & Jackson, D. D. (2011). *Pragmatics of Human Communication*. New York: Norton.

White, M., & Epston, E. (1990). *Narrative Means to Therapeutic Ends*. New York: W.W. Norton.

Winnicott, D. W. (1953). Transitional objects and transitional phenomena; A study of the first not-me possession. *The International Journal of Psychoanalysis*, 34(2), 89–97.

Winnicott, D. W. (1960). The theory of the parent-infant relationship. *The International Journal of Psychoanalysis*, 41, 585–595.

Winnicott, D. W. (1965). «Ego distortion in terms of true and false self». *The Maturational Process and the Facilitating Environment: Studies in the Theory of Emotional Development* (pp. 140–157). New York: International Universities Press.

Winnicott, D. W. (1967). «The mirror-role of the mother and the family in child development». In P. Lomas (Ed.), *The Predicament of the Family: A Psycho-Analitical Symposium* (pp. 26–33). London: Hogarth.

Winnicott, D. W. (1971). *Playing and Reality*. London: Tavistock Publications Ltd.

Winnicott, D. W. (1975). *Through Paediatrics to Psycho-analysis: Collected Papers*. London: Karnac Books.

Xinran (2010). *Message from an Unknown Chinese Mother*. New York: Scribner.

Acknowledgments

A.1

This book would have been impossible without the support and collaboration of so many people such that, almost certainly, I will forget to mention someone. I ask them to forgive me. I would like to at least highlight those who were of special relevance to me, in the process of writing, as well as in the work between Javier and Yao Lu.

To María Eugenia, director and coauthor of the book, I give my most sincere gratitude because she was able to see personal and professional virtues in me of which I was unaware. She knew how to help me explore them without pressuring me to do so, and instead invited me to discover them amidst the calmness and turbulence of the work experience we shared, contained and digested. Without a doubt, my professional path flourished with her support. My thanks goes to Mercedes Lozano Torrijos too, who was there when I needed her, and together, at times even through distant telephones, we digested uncertainties and anxieties.

To Mercedes Díaz-Salazar, one of my supervisors in training as a family therapist, I am also grateful. She was also encouraging in the discovery of my work as a co-therapist with her, and some of the interventions, like the one where Yao Lu and Javier conjure up a resonating past self on a chair, are directly related to her teachings and my experience with her.

To my roommates back then, David Martín Iglesias, Ángel Espadas Luengas, and Cristina Hernández Castillo, I give thanks for their respectful support without invading me with multiple questions, and for relinquishing our living room for me to use as a literary workshop for months. We transformed our apartment into a home, and nurtured the lasting bonds of a family between us.

I am profoundly grateful to the whole team of educators from both the Homes in Project *Sirio*, as well as to Teodoro Uría, psychiatrist and Balint group therapist. It would not have been possible for this work to take place without you. There are so many of you! Some of you might find yourselves in between the lines, and others more directly present in them, but you all formed part of the invisible ties in my network of supports.

My parents and sister, who since I was little encouraged me to write, knew not to insist too much once I shared this project with them. Your encouragement was also my inspiration. My brother-in-law also deserves much appreciation. He devoted significant time and creativity, and designed the artwork on the cover, capturing little Yao Lu and the Madrid skyline.

The English version of the book was no less of a task. I may have worked on it in every cafeteria in Brooklyn, over a period of five years. The translation got jump-started following an invitation to speak of the work at a Tuesday morning meeting at The William Alanson White Institute in 2014. Once I finished the initial draft, three people devoted significant time and energy to the project. By order, Thomas A. Frankel, my forest loving uncle, read and re-read the English draft offering priceless comments on metaphor use and translation to fit the meanings I was looking to convey. His mastery of both English and Spanish (and a few other languages) helped the book get to what it is today. He was the books' first editor once it was translated to English. Daniel Gensler, PhD, also read the book thoroughly, and turned it around with suggestions and edits before I thought it was humanly possible. Thanks to both of you. And Pascal E. Sauvayre, PhD, who was my clinical supervisor at the tail end of my training in Child & Adolescent Psychotherapy at The William Alanson White Institute, and who I continued to work with privately, took on the gargantuan task of becoming the professional editor. He corrected for style, read and reread metaphors, offered fitting ones, and helped make the complex theoretical concepts less opaque, which was a risk in translating them back into English. His mastery of these complexities has brought the book to its current form. I could not be happier having had their help.

My gratitude must also go to Carlos Avendaño, MD, PhD from the Department of Anatomy, Histology & Neuroscience of the Autónoma University of Madrid. He read the final draft in English closely, suggesting needed corrections.

And Anita Lanzi, PhD, also deserves ample thanks, for always listening and letting herself be moved. It moved me forward, on my path to become the kind of psychoanalyst I want to be.

But perhaps the one who should receive the most resounding gratitude is Yao Lu, who amidst the great uncertainties of her budding therapeutic relationship with Javier, with great courage, shared the emotional experiences of her world, and granted us permission to tell her story. It is through her and her relationship with Javier, and the other children like her and their relationships with their educators, that I learned to be the therapist I am today. They never ceased to surprise me and teach me, and for that I will be eternally grateful.

Tomás Casado-Frankel

A.2

I hear Tomás. Thank you, for knowing how to seize the opportunities with the hope, courage, and life you put into accompanying, and then writing, always eager to learn. Thank you Yao Lu. Thank you to our whole Team who, after 20 years, keep up the hopefulness and continue to gain knowledge for Yao Lu and others who are or will be different Yao Lus.

Thank you also …

To Taciana Fisac, Sinologue sister who searched for a symbolic and meaningful name for our "girl who made her way from a place far away …"

To Dr. Javier Avendaño, the first enthusiastic, and at the same time, incisive manuscript critic.

To Dr. Teodoro Uría, for his precise and accurate contributions.

To Alfredo Verdoy sj., historian and meticulous critiquing editor who read our manuscript one letter at a time, understanding and correcting.

To José Luis Olaizola, an experienced and prolific writer and a generous and kind neighbor, who openly read it generating interesting ideas.

To Vinyet Castro-Gil, always a thorough and kind editor (of the original manuscript in Spanish) from the lands of Galicia.

And to the great friends and as always generous sponsors of Sirio, in so many ways and forms: Marisefa Friberg, Rosa María de la Quintana, Ignacio Egea, Carmen Tartière, Carmen López Tartière, and Carlos Avendaño, who have also been paramount in making the publication of this book possible.

María Eugenia

And then one day:

Almost ten years after Javier and Yao Lu parted ways and after Javier had relocated to New York to continue his work and training, they met again. Javier and Yao Lu had agreed that he would let her know whenever he was back to visit, in case she wanted to meet up. For a long time they were unable to see each other. Life had taken over. They both occasionally heard about each other through the Project's team. And Javier always sent Yao Lu a text on her birthday. Yao Lu also reached out to Javier every so often with a "hello". Despite the vast physical distance, they remained connected.

And on one summer afternoon, when Javier was in Madrid on vacation, he reached out to let her know he was there:

Hi Yao Lu. I'm in Madrid and will be here until Sunday. I go back to New York on Monday. As promised, I'm letting you know. If you want to and have time, we could say 'hi'. It's okay if you can't. Sending you a hug.

"Ok. Let me know when and we'll meet. I have lots to tell you and we can talk like we used to!!"

They agreed on a time and place. And Javier ... Well, Javier was late! He got stuck in heavy traffic. But Yao Lu waited, and waited, and she patiently waited some more until he arrived.

They talked for close to three hours. Yao Lu caught Javier up on her life. There had been a few difficulties. Whose life doesn't have any challenges? Her family had grown and she had a few new children of her own.

Javier talked with Yao Lu and interacted with her young family. He watched her in her role as mother. Calmness threaded her narrative as she made sense of the past few years. That calmness soothed her children when they needed it too. Their affection for each other was clear. Something about Yao Lu was settled and different.

As they all walked down the street to a Chinese restaurant, her toddler crouched down, picked a dandelion, and ran up to show mommy. The flower had fought its way out through a concrete sidewalk. Yao Lu crouched down low, and under the bright sun, they looked at each other, and smiled in a moment of wonder.

Index

Note: Page numbers followed by 'n' denote endnotes

For Product Safety Concerns and Information please contact our EU
representative GPSR@taylorandfrancis.com
Taylor & Francis Verlag GmbH, Kaufingerstraße 24, 80331 München, Germany

www.ingramcontent.com/pod-product-compliance
Lightning Source LLC
Chambersburg PA
CBHW060257220326
41598CB00027B/4134